What If You Could
Skip *the* Cancer?

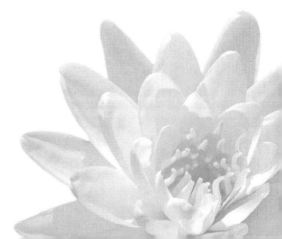

WHAT IF YOU COULD
SKIP *the* CANCER?

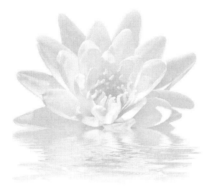

KATRINA BOS

FERNE PRESS

Summary: This book explains how honouring our unique perspectives on life can help to prevent cancer and other diseases before they ever appear.

Library of Congress Cataloging-in-Publication Data
Bos, Katrina (1969–)
What If You Could Skip the Cancer? / Katrina Bos – First Edition
ISBN-13: 978-1-933916-39-2
1. Healthy living. 2. Mental health. 3. Surviving cancer.
I. Bos, Katrina II. What If You Could Skip the Cancer?
Library of Congress Control Number: 2009927311

FERNE PRESS

Ferne Press is an imprint of Nelson Publishing & Marketing
366 Welch Road, Northville, MI 48167
www.nelsonpublishingandmarketing.com
(248) 735-0418

CONTENTS

To the divine spark in all of us

INTRODUCTION

In many great fables, there is often an eccentric outsider who helps the hero see their life more clearly. This outsider points out the pitfalls in the hero's life that the hero can't see because they have lived in the same village for their whole life. It takes the wisdom of the traveller to help them see their way out of their problems.

This is what happened to me.

I come from a long line of women who die from cancer at a young age. When I found lumps in my breast, I didn't want to become another link in that chain. I was desperate to find a different path. This is where my fable began. The eccentric outsider stepped into my life and everything I knew got turned upside down.

This is not a book about alternative medicine vs. conventional medicine. It is about ideas beyond both of these things. It is about beliefs and patterns that affect our health regardless of what treatment path we take.

It is about understanding how and why cancer comes to us in the first place. It is about looking at why it runs in families. It's about looking at some of our beliefs and habits, and wondering whether they are helping or harming us.

It is about learning from the people who got better—the "spontaneous healers." What sets them apart from those who die? What do they have in common? What if we could learn from them and make those same changes in our lives *before* we get sick?

What if we could skip the cancer?

CHAPTER ONE
THE BREAST LUMP

I was twenty-nine years old when I found the lump growing in my breast. I had had lumps before, but this one was different. It had been growing quite steadily for a while now and I didn't know what to do.

Finding a breast lump is no small matter for anyone, but I was from one of *those* families. You know, the families where all of the women die of cancer—my mom, her sister, their mom—one of *those* families.

At this point, medicine hadn't been able to help with whatever cancer the women in my family were dying from. It works for some people, but in my family, everyone had died—we were batting zero.

I remembered watching my mom four years earlier go through the chemotherapy, the radiation, the morphine, the whole thing, and I remembered knowing deep down that this wouldn't be my path.

And here I was lying in bed one night faced with this question: What other options are out there?

That's when serendipity stepped in.

The next day, as I was driving into town, my van suddenly lost control on a patch of ice. When I regained control and pulled over to the side of the road to catch my breath, a dark green Jeep pulled up beside me.

It was Jim—a man I had just met a few weeks ago. As luck would have it, he was someone who did healing work to help people with all kinds of diseases. He wasn't exactly a naturopath, but more like one of those gurus who was so grounded, he could see through your problems with a clarity that allowed him to get straight to the real issue. He was the kind of person that you climb to the top of the mountain to find in the movies.

I remember that the first time I met him, I asked him how old he was. Truthfully, if he had said that he was five hundred, I probably would have believed him—there was a wisdom about him that I had never seen before. It was easy to understand how he helped so many people.

"Hey stranger! Those were some fancy moves out there!" Jim said.

I sputtered something about not knowing why I had spun out because there wasn't any ice on the road. Then, as my brain started to slow down from my mishap, it dawned on me that I could ask Jim for help with my breast lump. But would he be able to help me? Was this the right path? As I sat there pondering this, Jim started telling me a story.

"You know, it's a funny thing. My friend's wife just died of breast cancer. What's weird is that they never asked me for help. The doctors said that there was nothing more that they could do for her. They knew that I did work with people, and yet they never even asked. Really weird. I just don't understand that."

"Yeah, people are weird, eh?"

"Yep. I mean, maybe I couldn't have helped her. Who knows? She might have died anyway. But you would think that they would have at least risked the possibility that I could've helped them out. I mean, all they had to do was ask!"

And then he smiled at me with this really kind, knowing smile—a smile that looked right down into your soul and woke you up to something.

As I looked at him, a thousand thoughts were going through my head. Is this my answer? Would this be a responsible thing to do considering my family history? What kinds of things might I have to do? Does he have time to fit me in?

Finally I decided.

"Jim, would you be able to take a look at a lump in my breast?"

Up until 1987, Jim had had a pretty normal life—married, three kids, picket fence, and all that. Then, one fateful day, he was carrying an extension ladder over his shoulder when he hit an overhead electrical wire. The electrocution did such extensive damage to his entire body that the doctors weren't sure whether he would live or die.

Amazingly, three days after the accident, Jim was walking and talking like nothing had ever happened. But he suddenly had an uncanny insight into people's illnesses and what they could do to get better. He was empathic—he could feel what other people were feeling. This was all very new to him, but he knew that he had to start using this gift to help people.

He started out just helping family and friends, and then the word spread. Soon, people were travelling from all over with all kinds of problems, from cancer to epilepsy to depression to marital problems.

What made him unique and invaluable to these people is that he saw their diseases and their problems "from the inside out." It was a completely different way of understanding why they were sick. He took the whole person into account—not just whatever part of their body was showing the illness.

I couldn't believe that he had shown up on this morning just at the right time. I couldn't believe that he was going to try and help me. I felt really lucky, and somewhat relieved, to have found a possible path.

Little did I know just how much these meetings with Jim would change my life, or how they would change the lives of my husband, my children, my sisters, my family, and just about everyone else I would ever come into contact with.

Everything that I thought I understood about cancer, happiness, and life would soon be turned upside down—never to be the same again. And it started with looking at how society views cancer and how that belief system affects our ability to heal.

OUR FEAR OF CANCER

Cancer has generally been perceived, understood, and treated in a certain way. It is seen as an intruder, an infection gone crazy, an external evil to be isolated, fought, and destroyed. We have even created a word for "things that cause cancer"—carcinogens. And we also have its opposite, anti-carcinogens—"things that fight cancer."

The problem is that looking at cancer from this perspective places cancer as the aggressor and us as its victims. All we can do is decrease the known carcinogens in our lives and increase the anti-carcinogens. This will arm us for the battle.

However, even with the billions of dollars spent on research each year, the fear of cancer is rising. Women of all ages are being told to go for mammograms regardless of their family history—just to be safe. We even hear about women who are so scared about the possibility of getting cancer that they have their breasts removed, hoping for peace of mind.

With all the information about eating right, exercising, and new treatments available, we should be feeling pretty good. But we aren't. We aren't feeling more secure. We are progressively becoming more afraid. Something is amok.

What are we missing? Why aren't we able to fight off the cancer? Why are our bodies so weak and undefended?

And what about the people who do survive? What about the ones whose bodies are able to beat the cancer? What about the stories of miraculous healings? Where do they fit into all of this?

What did they do differently from everyone else? How did they do it? What was different about them?

SPONTANEOUS HEALING

There are thousands of cases of spontaneous healings fully documented in medical journals. You expect to find stories of miraculous healings in alternative literature. But to find case studies in medical journals where there is scientific rigour is really inspiring.

There are stories of people who recovered from ulcers, all kinds of cancers, heart problems, asthma, AIDS, and more.

And these are just the reported cases that made it into the medical journals. Imagine how many more people had miraculous healings outside of the view of modern medicine, whose cases simply weren't reported to medical journals, or who had spontaneous remissions only to have the doctor decide that it must have been a misdiagnosis to begin with.

Each patient has their own story. There are women, men, and children. They are of different cultures and different religions. Some are blue-collar workers, some are professionals, and some are homemakers. Their diseases ranged from cancer to heart disease to massive injury from car accidents.

On the surface, they seemed to have nothing in common. The only common thread of their stories was that they were diagnosed as incurable—so incurable that the doctors figured that treatment was not an option anymore.

But the second thing that they had in common was that they survived. After the worst prognosis and no available treatment, they lived. And they didn't just continue living with their illness or injury. They healed. The disease disappeared.

This is no small thing. This cannot be ignored.

These people *healed*. And we are all made of the same flesh and bones as they are. We have that same ability inside of us. The question is, how do we do it?

SPONTANEOUS HEALING HAPPENS ALL OF THE TIME

Most of us consider spontaneous healing to be a miracle, a fluke, or an oddity. For someone who is facing a medical diagnosis of cancer, they generally figure that the best they can do is pray for a spontaneous healing. Often they hold little real hope.

We assume that the occurrence of such spontaneous healings is a rare thing.

But is it really?

What is it that happens when we cut our finger? What happens when we burn our mouth on hot soup? What happens when we stay out in the sun too long and get burnt to a crisp? When we exercise too long and strain our muscles? When everyone around us is getting "that flu that's going around," but we just have the sniffles for a day?

Our body is designed to heal itself. Spontaneous healing happens every day to every one of us.

In fact, when we say that a healing or regression was "spontaneous," it has nothing to do with unexpectedness or being miraculous. "Spontaneous" actually means that the healing came from the inside. It simply means that the process was generated from inside the body.

According to Collins Dictionary, spontaneous is defined as "occurring, produced, or performed through natural processes without external influence," or "arising from an unforced personal impulse; voluntary; unpremeditated."

This has nothing to do with strangeness, suddenness, or quickness, as we so often think when hearing the word "spontaneous." In fact, remissions are seldom sudden. They happen gradually over time. Spontaneous healings happen "through natural processes" and through "personal impulses." They are not all that miraculous, but actually quite natural.

And we already know this. Every time we put a bandage on a child's cut, our expectation is that the body will heal the wound and knit the skin back together. The bandage plays no real role in the healing, except for perhaps keeping the wound clean and making the child feel better.

Consider what happens if we break a leg. Why do we put a cast on it? Are there magical ointments under the cast that cause healing? Does the cast itself heal the break? No. The cast simply immobilizes the leg so that the body can do exactly what it is designed to do. Doctors fully expect and count on the fact that the bone will knit itself back together. They expect the muscles to heal and the skin to heal as well. The body's natural ability to heal is absolutely expected and counted on.

In fact, it is abnormal for the body *not* to heal. It is brilliant at healing. It is made for healing. Its goal is survival.

The Body is Designed for Regeneration

To understand this, we have to consider how our body works. Our body has an inherent intelligence that is continually healing and renewing itself.

The human body is different from a car. Once you build a car, the steel and the parts that were in it on its first day out of the factory stay with it until eventually the parts break down or the steel rusts. At this time, you take it in to the shop for repair.

But the human body isn't designed like that. It is constantly renewing itself. Individual cells are constantly being replaced. Your stomach cells, your skeleton, your bone marrow, your blood, your skin—they are all constantly doing an "out with the old and in with the new." They are constantly regenerating. The body you have today is not the same body that you had a year ago.

Imagine if our car could do that. What would that be like? We would never have to change the oil—it would constantly be cleaning itself. As we wore down the brake pads, they would simply keep regrowing. Our tires would never go flat from nail holes because as soon as a hole was detected, the car would automatically send a rubber-repair kit to fix it. If any rust started to form, the car would simply create new steel and paint in those spots. We would never have to go to the shop because our car would constantly be renewing and repairing itself. Sounds like science fiction? Well, that is exactly what our bodies do every day of our lives.

So, in theory, if something like a tumour were growing in our bodies, then the body's immune system would detect it and get rid of it. Most of the time, this is precisely what happens. The body disposes of growths, waste, and old cells all of the time. But if you have a chronic growth of some kind, like cancer, then something else is happening.

If you have a tumour in your body and it is still there after a year, then it is actually not the same tumour. All of the cells within it have been regenerated—out with the old, in with the new.

Think about this. That tumour is not the same tumour that was there a year ago. The body has been perfectly replicating it in order to keep it there!

Why would the body do this? Why would it regenerate a mutation like a tumour? Why would it regenerate itself improperly? Why wouldn't it recognize that the tumour doesn't belong?

What if there were a glitch in the body's intelligence that is in charge of regeneration? How else could it keep making the same mistake so perfectly and seamlessly that we wouldn't even realize that it wasn't the same tumour?

It would be like a factory worker on an assembly line who was given bad training or incorrect instructions. He would simply keep making the same mistake over and over again. He wouldn't know that anything was wrong until someone realized what was happening and his instructions were corrected.

Similarly, if there is a glitch in the body's intelligence, it must be rectified.

The question is: What is the glitch? And how do we fix it?

CHAPTER TWO
DEPRESSION

I had no idea what to expect at my visit with Jim. On one hand, I was excited and relieved to be looking into this breast lump and taking a step towards fixing it. But there was a fear too—a fear that I was opening up a Pandora's box that, once opened, I wouldn't be able to close.

There just seemed to be a sense that this wouldn't be any normal visit where you got your prescription or natural remedies and walked out. It just felt like more.

As Jim checked out the lump, he became very serious.

"What do you want to do?" he asked.

"I don't know. What do you mean?"

"I mean, what do you want? Do you want to get better?"

I wanted to reply with, "Of course I want to get better! What do you mean by that?" But there was something in the seriousness of his voice that made me pause and consider his question more seriously.

In my silence, he continued, "Do you know what the first thing was that Jesus asked people when they came to him for healings? It was 'Do you want to be healed?' This is the most important thing to know before you begin the process.

You have to realize that deep down not everyone wants to be healed from their diseases. It's not that they necessarily want to be sick. But they don't really want to be well either."

That didn't make any sense. Why wouldn't someone want to be better? Why would anyone want to be sick? I didn't get it. But there was something about this man that I trusted. And I really didn't trust easily. So I thought about his question and answered him.

"I want to get better."

"Okay. But you have to make a deal with me before I will work with you."

"All right."

"I don't think this lump is cancerous right now. But I don't like the way it is growing. I will give you two weeks of working with me. If there is no sign of improvement in that time, you must go to the doctor."

"Okay."

I didn't think that it would come to that. I really did feel like I was on the right path. I would honour my promise if I had to. But, deep down, I really hoped that I wouldn't have to.

The fact that Jim didn't believe that the lump was cancerous at that point gave me some peace of mind. But I didn't ever want it to become cancerous either. I had had many breast lumps over the years. Some had come and gone on their own, and others had been checked out by doctors. But for some reason this one seemed different. The way it grew was different. The way it felt was different.

The biggest difference between those lumps and this one was that now I had a daughter. Based on our family history, breast cancer was practically a 100 percent certainty for her. Maybe this lump was my opportunity to really understand my family's breast cancer legacy. I didn't know. But it felt like I was in the right place to find out what I needed to know—for me and for her.

Jim began talking about his experiences working with people with cancer. It didn't seem particularly directed at me. They were just stories about various people. They had different jobs, different body types, and different cultural backgrounds. But there were certain things that were very similar. They handled stress in very specific ways, they looked for love in very certain ways, and they were very often depressed.

As he talked, he would do various techniques on me. He never called them anything in particular. Some people would call what he did Reiki, energy balancing, massage, acupressure, hands-on healing, etc. But he never used the names that we would give them. He'd simply say that he asked for guidance as to what needed to be done and then he would do it. He wouldn't name it or even necessarily tell me what he was doing unless it was important that I knew. He would just go about his work, chatting to me about whatever happened to come up.

"This is what you need to learn how to do," he would say.

"What? Healing work?"

"No. Prayer. You need to learn how to ask for guidance, hear the answer; and then have the faith to do what you hear."

I didn't quite know what to do with that. First of all, it kind of got my hackles up. I had some issues with the church, faith, prayer, and all that. Second of all, I had never heard of waiting for an answer to follow. Our prayers are either answered or not, right? We sit and wait for the miracle. That's how it's supposed to happen. This was a new concept to me and so I just lay there in silence absorbing what he was saying.

Actually, I spent most of the time in our sessions just listening. Every so often, I would ask questions. But mostly, I just listened.

I listened because I had nothing to say. I had honestly come to the end of myself. I wasn't sure what the right way to live was anymore. I had done just what everyone (including myself) had expected of me. I got straight A's all through school. I went to university. I married a good man. I got a good job. Then I had babies. I even had two children, a boy and a girl—the million-dollar family! I worked on the farm. I made jam. I was president of the Parent-School Association. And yet, deep down, I was unhappy. I was restless.

But no one else would know it. According to society, I was very functional. I could balance family and work. I still attended family get-togethers with salad in hand and a smile on my face. My husband and I had a loving relationship. As far as society went, I was doing really well, considering I was able to do everything I did "happily," and I didn't even need Prozac to get me there!

But deep down, I was sad. Luckily, I was so busy that I didn't have the time or energy to worry about it. My marriage was still together and we were all healthy and happy. We should just feel blessed that we had food on the table and a roof over our heads. Right?

Suddenly, I started to cry. Tears just started pouring down my face. I had no idea why.

Jim just watched me kindly and smiled.

"What's wrong?"

"I don't know."

He looked at me for a moment and asked, "If you could do anything in the world, right now, what would it be?"

Without hesitation, I surprised myself by saying, "I want to go away."

"That sounds like a great idea! Why don't you? Tell you what! You could even stay here at the chalet. I won't be needing it for a while—you could have it all to yourself."

"I can't go away! I have two small kids. I have a husband, a farm—responsibilities! I can't just pick up and leave! That's crazy! It's impossible!"

He just looked at me, smiled, and said, "Well, you could die."

Die? Die? I could die? I had never thought of that. Then my family would really have to do without me—forever! I pondered that. Who would take care of them? Who would love them? Who would protect them? Who would make sure that they were happy?

But then I realized that someone would. They might struggle for a time. But they would get over it and they would get on with their lives. They might even thrive. It's always a shock to realize that the people you love would get along without you!

After these morbid and upsetting thoughts, the idea of going away for a couple of days didn't seem so ridiculous. Maybe a couple of days away to pray and ponder things and start to heal would be a good thing. Maybe I actually could do it.

And so, a couple of days later, my sister came to look after the kids. I packed a bag, kissed my husband and kids, and headed to the chalet for my first-ever personal getaway.

DISCOVERING DEPRESSION

I remember one time when I sent a really sick friend to go see Jim. After she left his place, she told me that all he did was talk about changing her diet and a few small things, but nothing amazing took place.

When I went to him for my next session, I asked him why he didn't help her.

He responded with, "Look Katrina. Until your friend admits to herself that she's depressed, there isn't anything that I can do for her."

I immediately started arguing the point that he could have done something. She had come all this way, she was really sick, etc.

He then looked at me and said slowly, "Would you like me to repeat that for you?"

"What?"

"Until she admits to herself that she is depressed, there isn't anything anyone can do for her."

Then he stared at me with that annoying grin on his face.

"Oh. You're talking about me again."

Convincing me that I was depressed was one of the first big hurdles. I thought, "Compared to whom?" I was absolutely one of the most upbeat people I knew. I didn't complain. I could always see the bright side. I was all about finding the silver lining. I was the one who made other people feel better. How could I be depressed? As far as society goes, I was pretty damn happy!

But that's the problem. We often look at ourselves only in comparison to others. I didn't think that I was depressed because everyone around me seemed unhappier than I was. But the real question was whether I was depressed compared to how happy I could be. How far below my own potential was I living?

Sure, I was pretty happy. I had everything that I wanted—a husband who loved me, great kids, security, and more comfort than most of the world's population has. I had nothing to complain about.

But was I satisfied? No. Was I excited about anything I was doing? No. Was I bored? Yes. Would I have liked my life to be different? Yes.

Hmm. I had a lot to think about.

HOW DOES THIS HAPPEN?

Imagine that you and your husband get married in your early twenties. You are bright, excited, and ready to take on the world. You both have the same dream—getting good jobs, buying a nice house, two cars, and having a gaggle of kids—the American Dream.

You both struggle at entry-level jobs for a time and then your husband lands the great job. There are chances at promotion, holidays, benefits, and income security! Soon after, babies start arriving. Because of your husband's great job, you have the opportunity to stay home with the little ones. And you do.

Being home is great, but raising children can also be really challenging at times. You have a network of friends and family that you find support in, which makes the challenge manageable.

And then you find out that you husband is being promoted in his job, which means a transfer. The kids are four and two years old. The move won't affect them all that much. It is only you that will lose your network of family and friends. But what can you do? What can you say? It would be selfish of you to ask him not to accept the transfer. And so you pack up your life and you go.

You find the new town, you have the struggle of being isolated, but eventually you make new friends, just in time to find out that another promotion and another transfer are coming. The kids are in school now. But this will be character building, right? And so you move again.

Now, I am not saying that this is a terrible lifestyle. (In fact, after living on a dairy farm for fifteen years, the idea of moving certainly holds some appeal for this gypsy!) The question is: What if you don't like moving? Do you say anything? Do you put your foot down and say no?

The likelihood is that, if you are the type of person who gets cancer, you probably don't say anything. You will keep moving with a smile on your face. You won't want to burden your husband. How can you complain when he has provided such a great life for you and your children? He has always been supportive of you. He is a good husband and a good father. It would be selfish to ask him to find a different job or ask that he not be transferred anymore.

Do you hear the arguments of the mind? None of these things has anything to do with your happiness. They have nothing to do with your state of mind or your heart's desires. After a while, your own heart's desires will simply go to sleep. They are irrelevant. You are stuck. You are in a prison that you can't see. You can't leave because you actually love your husband. But you don't feel that your opinions and feelings count for enough to really say something. Your own dreams are irrelevant. And so you stay quiet. And the depression deepens.

CANCER'S QUIET DESPAIR

Many people who get cancer live with a certain kind of depression for most of their lives. In fact, it moves a few steps past depression into despair.

This despair comes from a lifetime of not feeling that they could honour their truths. It comes from constantly doing things to make other people happy, trying to live up to other people's expectations, and always putting other people ahead of themselves.

Maybe you are a man who didn't follow your dreams because you had to provide for the family. Maybe you felt that you couldn't do all the things that you wanted to do because you had to live up to your parents' expectations or because it wouldn't look right in your community.

Maybe you are a woman who puts her family and everyone else's needs ahead of her own. Maybe you are acutely aware of how to keep peace in the tribe. You understand the importance of family groups and relationships. You are the peacemaker. And so, when a decision is to be made in the group, even if it is a decision that you would rather not go along with, you will likely concede.

Maybe you're the loving person who cares for your aging parents. Your parents are getting older and they are in need of care. They were always good to you and took care of you. You never even questioned whether or not you would take care of them in their old age. Of course you would.

All of these things are wonderful to do, so please don't think that I am saying that you shouldn't do them. But the question to ask is, "Can you do them and still pursue your own life and your own interests?"

Now, anyone who is *not* on the road to cancer would immediately say, "Of course you can. You have to. You'll go insane if you don't maintain a proper life balance."

But the rest of us have a different response.

We say things like:

"They really need me now. It's the least I can do."

"So what if I have to put my life on hold for a while."

"My needs are not as important as their needs right now."

And so on.

But what if there is something inside of you telling you that you are not happy about this? What if you are getting more and more tired and you are burning out? What if you are even starting to resent your loved ones for you having to give up your life? What if, deep down, you start to wonder how much longer they'll still be here?

These are very upsetting thoughts. They then cause even deeper guilt. What kind of monster are you? Now you definitely have to keep taking care of them. There's no way that you could send them to a nursing home!

The point is that you aren't being honest—not with yourself and not with them. This is a problem. There is great and wonderful guidance at your fingertips and you are shutting it out. And because of this, you are burning out. You are feeling resentful. You are feeling depressed and you just can't take it much longer.

THE ROLES WE PLAY

We have to look at this script that we are playing in our minds. We have been taught what we have to do to have a successful marriage, to be good parents, to be upstanding members of the community, etc.

We know the rules with every fibre of our being. We can barely separate ourselves from them.

We know what our roles are in the family. We know what a man or a woman is supposed to do, be, look like, and act like. Any deviation from that is going to cause problems. We know this deep down, even if we've never actually said it out loud.

We know as women what our role is in the tribe. We marry. We have babies. We are the caregivers. We bake for the bake sales. We throw the birthday parties. We do the Christmas shopping. We entertain and make Jell-O salads for the family picnics.

We know as men what our role is. We work. We provide. We play ball with the kids. We drive the kids to hockey. (These days, we might even wash dishes and change diapers too.)

If we follow the rules, our lives will be complete. Everything will be perfect. Right?

But it isn't. There is a rumbling deep down that says that we want more. There are desires and thoughts and dreams that don't dare come up because there are so many people depending on us staying exactly the same. If we suddenly changed, it would create havoc in so many people's lives. And so we keep the inner rumblings quiet.

But it doesn't work. After a while, other things start to fester. Resentment starts brewing towards the very people that we are caring for. Do you know why? Because they are human. They will not show nearly enough appreciation for what we do because they have no idea how much we are giving up in order to do what we do for them.

But you are a really nice person. It is not sensible to be resentful towards your family. They are everything to you. So you ignore the resentment too. It just can't be happening.

But as you bury more and more of the feelings that you are having, you start to feel further and further away from everyone that you love. The problem is that it is only honest communication that creates close bonds with other people. But you can't be totally honest with anyone. You wouldn't know where to start.

You are honest in the way that society expects you to be honest. You don't lie about anything in day-to-day life. But your feelings? Your dreams? They are kept under wraps.

No One Knows

After a while you start to feel very alone. But no one else knows. No one knows how you are feeling. In fact, most of the time, you don't know how you are feeling. You are just going through the motions of life. You truly love your family deeply. But it just isn't enough.

But how could you complain? You have more than most. You are just having a bad day. This feeling will pass. Maybe you're just hormonal.

But it doesn't pass. Days, weeks, and years go by. You still have the good life. You are doing all the right things. But nothing really feels like it's yours. Something is missing. You can't name it. Maybe you're crazy. Maybe you are expecting too much.

The problem is that the less you talk about it with anyone, the more you feel alone. It's like there is no one in the world that knows how you really feel. No one knows your dark little secret. And you don't want to tell anyone because it just seems crazy, you already feel guilty about it, and there's nothing anyone can do about it anyway.

So you stay quiet.

And the depression deepens.

Chapter Three
The Mind/Body Connection

*The greatest discovery of every generation is that human beings
can alter their lives by altering their states of mind.*
Albert Schweitzer, MD

My mom had always been terrified of getting breast cancer. And she had been terrified for her girls. She had three daughters. I was the eldest.

Some of the saddest days of my childhood were the days after Mom would go for her yearly mammograms. Each year, she would go and have her breasts flattened like pancakes in order to see if the family inheritance of cancer was going to be passed down to her this year or if we got to wait until next year. (At that time, it was only women in families like mine that were told to go regularly.) Since my mom had large breasts that had a lot of normal lumps in them, the test was really painful for her.

For days after that, she would wait for the results. She didn't openly share her worries with us—she wouldn't want to upset us. But we always knew. Sometimes the results would come back and there would be a shadow. Maybe she would have to go back in so they could check it again or do a biopsy.

I felt so sorry for my mom those days. From the time she had to go for the test till the time that she received the results, it was like her life just stood still. She couldn't think about anything else until the tests were finalized, one way or another.

My mom first got sick when I was in my third year at university. It had started as breast cancer and then metastasized to the bones. She got pretty sick pretty fast. Initially, the doctors said that the cancer had progressed too far and it was so widespread that there was little that they could do. They could start with chemotherapy but they didn't want us to get our hopes up. They gave her six months to live.

We didn't know what to do. There had to be other options besides the doctors' prognosis of six months. There had to be more that we could do than just sitting by her bedside feeling helpless.

Then I remembered hearing about some guy who had laughed himself out of some horrible disease. It wasn't cancer, but it was something. How could I find out about him? Back in the late 1980s when my mom got sick, there were no self-help sections in the bookstores and the internet didn't exist. This kind of information was out there, but it wasn't necessarily easy to find.

So, I went to the psychology building on my campus and started knocking on doors. As each door opened, I asked them whether they had ever heard of some guy who had used laughter to heal himself. It took a while, but I finally found someone who recognized the story as that of Norman Cousins. I soon found his book, *Anatomy of an Illness*, which began my quest to understand the link between the mind and disease.

Norman Cousins had had a terribly debilitating bone disease that caused him constant pain. After no luck with medicine, he locked himself in a hotel room with a huge stack of slapstick comedy movies. He spent the entire weekend laughing himself silly and walked out pain-free. He spent the rest of his life studying the connection between the mind and the body and understanding the mind's ability to heal the body.

I raced back to Toronto where my mom was in the hospital to show her what I had found. We didn't have to accept the doctors' diagnosis. We could find another way. Other people had done it. There was hope!

My dad and sisters and I were all very hopeful and excited. But Mom just smiled at us politely. Maybe it was the cancer. Maybe it was the medication. I don't know. But it was like she just couldn't hear me. She was ready to go this route regardless of the prognosis. Honestly, after losing her mom and older sister to cancer, I think that she had been sort of waiting for this to happen her whole life. And now it finally had. For her, it was almost a relief. The wait was over. There wasn't anything to fear now. The worst had finally happened. There wasn't any energy left to fight it now—just quiet resolve that this was simply how it was going to happen.

But my dad and sisters and I were on a new track. We had found hope. We knew that there were other options than the ones that had been offered to Mom. We soon tracked down any information we could find about the connection between the mind and illness.

Mom tried her best with whatever we found that might help her. We found books written by Bernie Siegel, Deepak Chopra, Wayne Dyer, and Carl Simonton—doctors who were connecting the mind with the body and working with people with cancer. When she couldn't focus on reading books, we would find books on tape and she would listen to them on a headset. We found special teas and herbs for her to try. We read to her. We meditated with her. We went to seminars. We tried everything that we could find.

For the most part, I think Mom just went along with us. She did the reading and listened to the tapes. She did the visualizations and all that. And I hope that she had some hope at some time. But I think that she was pretty tired. I think that all the new ideas were overwhelming to her because of the cancer and all the medication that she was on. But she tried and was very patient with us.

Mom lived for another three years in almost constant treatment in and out of the hospital, including many kinds of chemotherapy and radiation. In those four years, she saw all three of her daughters get married and she celebrated her twenty-fifth wedding anniversary. She died two weeks after my youngest sister got married. My other sister and I were both pregnant with our first babies, the next milestone we were hoping that she'd make. But Mom never knew.

That was my first real awakening to the whole concept of the mind/body connection. After that, I read anything that I could find on the topic. I told anyone who would listen about the power of the mind to heal the body. But I hadn't really had to put it to the test. Sure, I had had some headaches that I had gotten rid of using relaxation and meditation, but nothing terribly serious.

But now I had a lump in my breast. I was faced with really walking my talk. It is one thing to believe these things in theory. It is quite another thing to be married with two small children sitting on the edge of your own mortality.

There was a time, not that long ago, that for scientific purposes, there was a clear split between the mind and the body. The body was physical and the mind was just thoughts. The body and mind worked independently of each other. So when something was wrong with the body, the mind was ignored. And when something was wrong with the mind, the body was ignored.

But this is not so any longer.

The problem was that looking at the physical body alone wasn't working. There were too many things that didn't make any sense. There were people surviving incurable diseases that shouldn't have. There were others dying of diseases who should have been all right.

It was like they were missing information. The picture was just too small. Important facts were being ignored.

Many doctors started noticing other things about their patients. They started noticing that many people who had heart attacks were Type A personalities. They noticed that many people who got cancer were people-pleasers. They noticed that people who were stressed out and worried tended to get ulcers.

So, they started looking at other non-physical aspects in their patients. What did they think about? What did they believe? How involved were they in the process of healing? How many questions did they ask? How many loved ones did they have around them? Did they have interests? Were they worried about other people's opinions? Were they depressed? How much "fight" was in them?

They found that people who survived often expressed their emotions more freely, weren't so concerned with other people's opinions, had faith in something bigger than themselves, and took control in their lives.

Slowly, these bits of information started finding their way into the medical journals. Eventually, this information started becoming large enough quantities of data that it couldn't be ignored if we were to understand why certain people lived while others died.

Nowadays, the basic concept that the mind is connected to the body is widely accepted. We all accept the placebo effect, that is, if we believe that the treatment we are receiving will help us, there is a high probability that the body will respond positively, even if the treatment itself is not inherently beneficial. And similarly, if we believe that the treatment will harm us, then the body will respond negatively.

Positive mental imagery is used regularly with athletes to help overcome blocks in their performance. If they can ski down the mountain course in their minds perfectly, then there is a high likelihood that they will repeat that perfect performance at the competition.

The effects of relaxation and meditation on the body are measurable with biofeedback machines. We know that stress adversely affects our immune system, our nerves, our heart, our digestion, etc.

We know that the connections between the mind and body are numerous. But what other connections are we still missing? And how do they relate to cancer?

Chapter Four
Getting Away

And so, off I went to the chalet.

And I slept. I think on the first day I slept for fourteen hours. To sleep until I woke up was such a novel thing for me. When you become a mother, it seems that you are always being woken out of a deep sleep. First they are babies waking up in the night. Then they are having nightmares, or they are sick, or they are potty-training. A decent night's sleep becomes a rare and wonderful thing.

Even just getting married disturbs your sleep. You are sleeping with another person, you have different schedules, you've got to get up for work, you have different alarms and nightly rituals, etc. Oftentimes, you don't even have your own personal schedule because your schedule is defined by everyone else's schedule. When does your husband get up? When do the kids have to get up to catch the bus or get to hockey practice? To get away and go to bed when I was tired and then wake up when I was rested was truly magical.

Once I did wake up fully rested, I felt like a completely different person. My eyes were clear, the sun was shining, and my mind was calm. I had a chance to think.

I had a chance to think because there were none of the normal distractions at the chalet. There was no TV, no telephone, no email, nobody needing me, nobody expecting anything from me. There was just me, alone with my thoughts.

Being alone, I was forced to slow down and listen to myself. I couldn't use anyone else as an excuse for not listening. It was just me.

I thought of Mom. I thought about my life. I thought about my kids. I thought about cancer. I thought about what I really wanted in life. It was like every thought that was normally trying to eke its way into my busy life was taking this chance to be heard.

When the thoughts got to be too much, I would journal. I just wrote everything down completely unedited. I rambled on for hours and hours, not with the intention of ever reading it again, just to get the thoughts out of my head.

I also spent a lot of time praying. That's what Jim had said that I had to do. I really trusted him, and he had said that prayer was the way through.

So, I prayed. I prayed during the day. I prayed every night before bed. I asked that the lump get smaller, that it be gone by morning—things like that. Strangely enough, the lump never was gone by morning. This really frustrated me. I figured, "Isn't that how the miracle is supposed to happen? I pray, I really mean it, and the lump goes away. That's the deal, right?"

But then I wondered, "Why do I really want it to go away?" Is it for the story? Do I just want to be able to yell from the rooftops that I prayed and my lump went away? Is this just some kind of ego trip for me? That was a disturbing thought.

Actually, I had many disturbing thoughts. I thought a lot about my mom and her ordeal with cancer. That brought up all kinds of emotions and frustrations that I thought that I had dealt with, but apparently hadn't.

I thought about an article I had read where they asked you to name six things that you love to do. I couldn't name one. I was sure that I had once loved to do things. But it had been so long that I didn't know what they were. I knew what my husband and kids liked to do. But what made me happy? I didn't even know where to start.

There was something wrong with that. What was I doing with my life? Why was there nothing in my life that actually brought me joy? I was thankful for my husband and kids and I loved them with all of my heart. But I wasn't happy.

I spent three days at the chalet. I was rested. I had prayed. I had journalled. I had pondered many things. By the time I left, it seemed like the lump was smaller. I liked to think so anyway. But it certainly wasn't gone. No miracle had occurred (except for the fact that I had actually gone away by myself for three whole days!).

There have been times in my life when a part of me silently wished that I had a broken leg. I'd have to spend weeks and weeks in a hospital where all I could do all day was rest and read the mountain of books that I never had time for.

Now, for anyone who has spent a lot of time in the hospital, we know that it isn't all sunshine, roses, and great reading time.

But it is interesting to note why this fantasy appeals to me—I get to rest. I get to read. I get to spend time with myself without any of the responsibilities and stresses of everyday life. It would seem that these things are what my heart is truly longing for—not the broken leg.

I never had time to just sit around and relax. There are so many pressing needs and things to do. And would it really make a difference? All the stresses of my life would still be there when I got back.

Stop Pedalling

A friend of mine always said that life was like being on a bicycle: she had to perpetually keep pedalling or else the world would stop turning.

What do we think would happen if we stopped pedalling? What if we just took a break for a while? This could take the form of a weekend away by ourselves. Or perhaps it is just stopping everything for a while. We could stop cleaning the house and planning the meals, or take a break from driving Johnny to hockey and Sarah to piano lessons and pressing our husband's shirts after everyone else goes to bed.

What if we just stopped and rested for a while?

We could stop listening to the news and staying informed. We could take a back seat in business meetings and let other people step forward.

We could stop worrying about what other people thought. We could simply smile or chuckle when someone was mean or condescending to us.

We could just relax.

What is the worst thing that would happen?

Our house might get messy. Our family might live on cereal and toast (or possibly choose to cook something). Our kids might find other ways to get to their extracurricular events or just take a year off and let everyone relax after school.

We might not be up to date on who is bombing whom, how many homicides Toronto is up to, or what the current argument is about in the House of Commons.

Strangely enough, it wouldn't really be so bad. We could live with this. If this is the worst case, taking a rest might just be worth it.

But the actual results would likely be better than that.

We would be relaxed, centred, and peaceful. Wouldn't that be a greater benefit to us and our families in the end? Not to mention what it would do for our state of mind and our health.

The Masks We Wear

The problem is that we are normally walking around utterly exhausted. And it isn't just our lifestyles that are exhausting. The reality is that as we pedal and pedal, we also uphold certain personalities to the world. We must portray a certain face depending on whom we are with. Carl Jung called them our personas—the masks that we wear for the rest of the world. Maintaining these masks is exhausting.

There is the face that we wear for our spouse—the face that hides any of the thoughts and opinions that we don't want them to hear or know about.

There is the face that we wear for work—the face that allows us to become exactly who we need to be to do our job in the best way that we can. No problems from home. All smiles for the boss. Coffees all around. Everyone's star employee.

Then there is the face that we wear for our children. This one can be a pretty true reflection of our real selves. But not always. We don't want our kids to know if we are depressed or struggling or mad or frustrated. We don't want them to know if we are worried about them or struggling with what we should do differently to help them. We want them to remain children and not be burdened with our adult problems. So, on goes the mask.

Then there is the face for the in-laws. And what about the face for the neighbours, and the teachers, and the cashier at the supermarket, and so on.

Keeping up these masks is exhausting. Some of them are necessary, but others could probably be taken off more often. Regardless, they can be exhausting to maintain.

Plus, we can't always tell where the mask ends and we start. To be healthy, we need to take the masks off regularly, hang them on the wall, and just be ourselves.

But when we are surrounded by kids and spouses and people all day long, the masks end up being on for so long that we soon forget where the mask ends and we start. We start to think that we are the person that we portray to our spouses and children. We start to identify with the role that we are playing. We lose track of the real person inside.

This is why, once in a while, it is so important to get away and be alone. When we get away, there is no one to see the masks. One by one, we can hang them on the wall and just be ourselves.

For me, getting away the first time was almost unnerving. It had been so long since I was "just me," I almost felt naked—like those masks protected me from something. It was very strange.

WE AREN'T ALONE

It is important to note that many great thinkers, philosophers, seers, and prophets also took regular sabbaticals. Time in the desert was a requirement for Jesus. There was Buddha sitting under his Bodhi tree. Carl Jung had a special cabin where he would go for days to get away from the hubbub of life. Henry David Thoreau actually moved to a little cabin in Walden Woods so that he could understand society more objectively.

They didn't do this because they were of divine birth or something. They did this because they needed to, and to be an example—for us to understand that we need time away, sometimes simply to absorb and percolate the changes that are going on in our lives.

They needed to put down their roles and just be themselves. They needed the space and time to connect with their innermost thoughts and dreams. And so do all of us.

Getting away and having alone time is not just a luxury. It might be an absolute necessity for our mental and physical health.

CHAPTER FIVE

THE PECKING ORDER

This above all: to thine own self be true.
William Shakespeare

"So how did you enjoy the chalet?" Jim asked.

"It was nice—very peaceful. Thanks for letting me use it."

"No problem. Did you learn anything?"

I wasn't sure what to tell him. I told him about journaling and praying and sleeping and the surprising challenges of being alone. But, truthfully, I was really disappointed that some kind of miracle didn't occur. I didn't have time for this lump situation to go on for too much longer. How many times was I going to be able to desert my husband and kids—and to have nothing really come of it? I had to get well sooner than later.

But I couldn't tell him this. It sounded wrong or arrogant or selfish or something. Who was I to tell him that I deserved a miracle? Who was I to be sad because my prayers weren't answered? I was happy enough that he was willing to work with me. I wasn't about to start complaining that the process wasn't working or just working too slowly to suit me.

But Jim was one of those people that you couldn't lie to. He saw right through me anyway. I wanted to say something, but I couldn't admit to him what I was thinking. And so, instead of speaking, the tears started to flow.

As he watched me cry, he asked me a question.

"Do you really want to live?"

Again with the strange questions! Why would he ask me that? Of course I wanted to live! I had everything to live for. I was married to a great guy. I had two young, healthy kids. I had my whole life ahead of me. I was only twenty-nine years old! Why wouldn't I want to live?

"Yes. I want to live."

But I said it quietly, tentatively. The way he asked me caught me off guard. This wasn't a flippant question. He was very serious in wanting to hear the answer. And it had to be absolute truth. But I really thought that I did want to live. I wasn't lying. I thought that was what I wanted. Later, I would realize that I wasn't really aware of how I actually felt.

Jim pulled out a piece of paper and a pencil.

"One of your biggest problems is that your pecking order is all screwed up. Not just you—most people."

"What's a pecking order?"

"Your pecking order is how you prioritize in your life, where you take your 'orders' from. It's like a pack of dogs. Every dog knows who the alpha male is. All decisions come down to him. In politics, there is a hierarchy of command that is followed. The president is supreme. The vice president is next. And so on.

"We all have an internal pecking order. We default command to certain people or powers in our life. There are things that take first priority and second priority and then everything else happens if there is time.

"The question for you is: What does yours look like?"

I thought about it and then scribbled on the paper something like:

Aaron and Taylor

Wayne

Farm

Family

Friends

In-laws

Neighbours

Jim smiled. "Wow! This is a great pecking order—if breast cancer is your goal in life."

"WHAT?"

It was actually hard to be offended by him. He always said things with a little twinkle in his eye that let him say all kinds of things like that without you taking it personally.

"All I'm saying is, if you want to get breast cancer, you definitely are on the right track!"

"Are you trying to tell me that it is wrong to take care of my kids and family? That I have my priorities mixed up because I am trying to be a good mother and wife? How does that make sense?"

He just sat there and smiled at me. So I gave in.

"Okay. What's my pecking order supposed to look like, then?"

"Well, it depends what you are going for. If your goal is health and happiness, your pecking order must look like this:"

God
Self
Spouse
Kids
Everyone and everything else
(job, family, friends, neighbours, etc.)

This didn't compute at all for me. I was a young mother and wife. How in the world could I put my spouse, let alone me, ahead of my kids? I wondered if this guy was off his rocker. And what in the world did this have to do with cancer?

"How can I put my spouse above my kids?" I asked. "My kids have way more needs than my husband does. They are dependent on me. He is a full-grown adult."

"The reality is that it was the two of you who brought those kids into the world. The best thing you can give them is two happy parents with a loving, healthy relationship. If you ask any child of divorced parents what they would want most, their answer will almost always be that they want their parents to be happy and back together. And let's face it, you and your husband are setting the biggest examples for them in their future relationships. That is a pretty important gift to be giving them as they go out into the world!"

Okay. I could buy that. But part of my frustration in my marriage was that my husband never had time for me. He was constantly working on the farm. And there truly was a ridiculous amount of work for him to do. He worked fourteen to sixteen hours a day and he still couldn't get ahead of it all. I even worked on the farm to help him. But the work just never seemed to get any less. And in the end, any chance at real intimacy or the fun that we used to have when we were dating was long lost in exhaustion and not having enough time.

"But what if his pecking order is out of whack? I am sure that I am not high on his list of priorities!"

"That will be a problem for him. No man who puts work ahead of his wife and family will have a happy marriage. It just doesn't work. But your husband's pecking order isn't your biggest problem."

He looked at me with those twinkling eyes again and that all-knowing smirk on his face.

"Where are you and God on your list?"

The reality is that the day I got married, my husband ended up on the top of the list. I was thrilled to have found someone that I loved and who actually loved me back! I would have done anything to keep my marriage happy.

Then when the kids were born, they had so many immediate needs. They took the top spot. In the day-to-day running of things, my kids ruled my life. But for the big decisions, Wayne was on top. This meant that if his dream was to own and run a successful dairy farm, then that is what I wanted too. It meant that if there was anything at all that I could do to make his life easier, then that's what I was going to do.

The result of this was that eventually, I had no life of my own. I used to call myself Wayne's "beck-and-call girl." If he needed me in the barn, then out I went with kids in tow or in a backpack carrier. I did the bookwork. I cleaned the house, made the meals, took care of the kids, etc. Plus I helped him in the barn or in the field whenever he needed me.

Now, there was nothing wrong with helping out my husband. But did I really *want* to do this? Was this my calling? Is this why I was put on this earth? The truth was that I didn't want to be a farmer's wife. But it was so clearly my husband's dream, I couldn't break it to him. So then the question was, why didn't I think that he could handle my truth? Or was I simply too afraid to find out?

Honestly, I was terrified of losing him. I had always had pretty poor self-esteem. The fact that I actually found someone who loved me was completely unbelievable to me. And deep down, the fact that he loved me defined me as a lovable person. I was someone worth loving.

Hollywood does a great job portraying "non-marriage material." They are always ugly, fat, or impossible to live with. No one wants to be that person—the person that no one would want to marry. So, the fact that Wayne wanted to marry me pulled me out of that category! Whew!

I now know that this is a ridiculous notion! I absolutely could not look at all of the married people I know and say that they are all more good-looking or kind or smart than my single friends. It is absolutely a Hollywood myth!

But I didn't know that then. So what did that mean to me and my life? It meant making sure that my marriage survived at all costs. Because if Wayne woke up one day and decided that being married to me just wasn't worth the effort, then I would be "non-marriage material" again and therefore unlovable. I couldn't live with that!

And so, in order to keep my marriage "happy," I told him what he wanted to hear. When he asked my opinion, sometimes I shared my truth. But often, I didn't even know what my truth was. I was so accustomed to trying to anticipate what he wanted and what he wanted to hear, I wasn't even connected to my truth anymore.

The funny thing is that before we got married, I was quite opinionated and independent. That was the person that he married. (In fact, my in-laws would argue that I still am and always have been!)

But after getting married, I turned into someone else. I became who my mom was in her marriage. I became a subservient and friendly doormat. (Interestingly enough, my mom did the same thing. She was very independent and fun before she got married. She lived with girlfriends, smoked, drove a sports car, and travelled the world. Then she got married and became just like her mom.)

It's like a magic switch goes off inside of us as soon as we get married, and we revert to our family's status quo.

So somehow, I was going to have to put myself and God at the top of the list and drop my husband down a couple of rungs. I was sure that he wasn't going to like it. But that's one of the benefits of having a breast lump—it gives you the courage to try something new without people arguing—much.

GETTING YOUR PECKING ORDER STRAIGHT

One of the challenges of putting ourselves so high on the pecking order is that it seems to be the opposite of what we are taught.

We are taught to be selfless. We are taught to put the needs of others before our own. Not only are we supposed to do this, we look up to, praise, and honour people who do it.

And so, when we get married and have children, putting the needs of our spouse and children first is a natural thing. This is how we are the best partner and parent that we can be. And we want to be the best we can be. We want our partner to always love us and we want to do a good job. We want our children to love us. And we want to give them the best start in life that we can. And giving everything we have over to them seems to be the best and surest way to do that.

But imagine that there is an error in this train of thought. Not that it is totally wrong. But it isn't complete. There are important pieces missing. And those pieces make all the difference in terms of our health and true happiness.

THE SACRIFICIAL PERSONALITY

Jim once told me that there was a pattern among many women who get breast cancer. They tend to be the ones who never say no to anyone, are always smiling, never ask for help, and always try to please others.

I wasn't surprised. Not only did I recognize it in myself, I certainly saw it in my mom, my sisters, and throughout our family. Then, when I talked to other women who had breast cancer, it was almost a guarantee that they too recognized the pattern in themselves and their families.

There are those of us who were raised with a very specific notion of what the ideal woman is. We know how she acts in marriage. We know how she treats her kids. We know how she acts in the community. For those of us with breast cancer in our families, we know all this because our ideal role model was our mother.

She was always there for us. She was everything to our fathers. She was selfless in relationships. She put everyone's needs ahead of her own. When she got sick, there was a never-ending parade of visitors and well-wishers. When she got really sick, all of her kids would sit by her bed-side because there was nowhere else that they could be. Their husbands often took early retirement to care for them, spending night after night sleeping in uncomfortable reclining chairs in the hospital.

Who wouldn't want to be loved that much?

Why wouldn't we emulate someone like that?

Why wouldn't we do everything that we could to be just like her?

But what if her life wasn't as rosy on the inside as it seemed to us from the outside? What if there were sacrifices that she was making to be the wonderful woman that we knew? What if those sacrifices contributed to a quiet depression that she couldn't share with anyone? What if that quiet depression caused a suppressed immune system? What if all those things that she took to heart and cared about so much over the years actually might have contributed to her cancer?

And cancer candidates aren't always wives and mothers. They can also be the ones who give up decades of their lives caring for elderly parents—never saying no, always being the ones that everyone can count on.

So what is so wrong with that? What is wrong with caring for others and being dependable and loving?

The problem is that we do it at the expense of ourselves and our own needs. Our own life is essentially put on hold while we care for everyone else. Our own needs and dreams are irrelevant. We tell ourselves that one day we will be able to pursue our dreams. But after a few decades, we can't even remember what our dreams were.

Our lives are simply run by caring for the needs of other people—which is fine, except that we end up having no control or say in our own lives.

A Sense of Control in Their Lives

The most well-documented change that spontaneous healers make before they get better is a shift to "personal autonomy," or taking control of their lives. It is a shift of power, or an awareness of a person's own right to live as they want to. It is an inner shift—something not easily explained or easily accomplished.

Some who went home to die were not told the truth about their prognosis, at the request of their family. With the news that they were going to be all right, they made an inner promise that they would never be sick again. They were going to really enjoy and love life! And they did.

For others who were told their prognosis, the news of their impending death caused them to decide to really live life to the fullest. They got rid of chronic stressors in their lives. They made love as often as possible. They drank beer with their friends and picked up hobbies that they had long forgotten about.

For others, the idea of truly facing death made them suddenly wake up to something. Maybe they had just been gliding through life up until this point. Maybe they had been relying on the opinions and guidance of others, not truly taking the reins in their own lives. But this was their wake-up call. They suddenly "came home." They were going to run the show from now on.

The "I Am" Experience

Rollo May called this inner shift the "I am" experience.

The "I am" experience is that moment when you suddenly realize that you are an individual person and that your perspective matters. This seems like a logical thing to believe. But many of us live a long time catering to the opinions and needs of everyone around us, with our own hopes, opinions, and thoughts coming second if they're even there at all.

The "I am" experience is when you start to see the world through your own eyes and stop wondering how everything would look to your spouse or your family or your friends or your colleagues. First, you digest whatever comes to you through your own filters and make your own decisions, and then you consider what someone else would think about it later, if at all.

Once this happens and you are able to truly live through your own experience, the changes you make have a significant effect on your life.

But just having the shift isn't enough. It is not the solution. It is just the first step. Without it, nothing else matters. It is the necessary foundation for starting to heal for good. It is the first thing that you must do in order to find out who you are and what you're all about.

It is the difference between joining the gym because other people are doing it or think that it would be a good idea for you, and consciously making a decision to join a gym because it is something that you really want to do—something that you would really enjoy.

When you join for the first reason, when (and if) you go, you will tend to do it mindlessly, just putting in the required time so that you can say that you did it. But your heart won't be in it. You will have just filled some time with the "appropriate" behaviour.

But when you join because it is something that you truly want to do, you will look forward to going. You will meet people with similar interests. You will feel great and enjoy every minute of your time there. It won't be a dreary workout. It will be a fun and uplifting experience with your body and mind.

Some survivors started doing yoga after they were diagnosed. Did the yoga cure them? We don't know. The question that we really want to ask is, "Why did they start doing yoga?" Did they do it because someone told them that it would be a good idea? Did they do it because they read a story about someone else that did yoga and got better?

Or did they start doing yoga because they chose to—because they were following the little voice inside that said, "Do yoga. This is on your path to wellness. Take care of yourself. You matter enough to do this for you."

The same goes for changing your diet. Some people have reported curing cancer after becoming a vegetarian or changing their diet to macrobiotic or raw foods.

Again, the question that has to be asked is, "Why did they do it?" Was it because they read about it in a book and figured that was what they should do too? Did someone tell them to do it and they just followed that person's advice?

Or did their little voice say that it was a good idea? And then, did they feel that their well-being was important enough to rock the boat a little at home and start eating differently even if it might pose some challenges for the family's dinner time?

It's like trying to lose weight or quit smoking or stop drinking. When you make the decision from an inner place and you are doing it for you, you have a much better chance of succeeding. But if you are losing weight to look good for other people or you are quitting smoking because other people think you should, the success rate is pretty dismal.

The "I am" shift must happen first. It creates the new solid foundation. It is the core of getting our pecking order straight. After that, decisions are made from the inside out. Changes we make have the chance to have great effect.

If we want to be healthy, we have to be sure of who's in charge.

Chapter Six
Inheritance vs. Genetics

*We are not the stuff that abides, but patterns that
perpetuate themselves.*
Norbert Weiner

The scary thing is that my mom had been just like me. She did everything for everyone. You never really knew how she felt because all that mattered to her was that you were happy. She was a "good" wife, a "good" mom, and a "good" friend. And she always had a smile on her face. But now, looking back at her as an adult, I wondered if she was ever really happy deep down. Her smile seemed to mask tears a lot of the time. She seldom expressed her emotions unless they were positive ones. And even when she was upset, her first concern was that her distress wasn't upsetting you.

When I was about seven years old, I remember going into the kitchen because I had heard the phone ring and then my mom scream. As I walked into our little seventies-era kitchen with the tacky wallpaper and the wrought-iron kitchen table, I could see my mom in the corner slumped over in the chair crying. I just stood back for a minute because I had never seen my mom upset before. I didn't know what to do.

She had just found out that her older sister, Ruby, had died of cancer. Their mom had also died of cancer, so the fear had always been there for them. I guess Aunt Ruby had been sick with the cancer for a while. I was too young at the time to know. But now she had died. All I could hear was Mom quietly saying "no, no, no" into the phone.

I must have moved or made a noise, because Mom suddenly looked up and saw me there. She called me over and gave me a big hug. She tried to stop crying so that she could make sure that I wasn't upset by what was going on. She was like that. Her sister had just died of a disease that had taken every woman in her family, but she was concerned that I would be upset by her being upset. But that was Mom.

And I wanted to be just like her. Everyone loved her. She was one of those people who just lit up the room when she walked in. She was an elementary school teacher with bright red hair and crazy earrings. She had a ukulele band and was always laughing. She had a thousand friends. You had to like her. She was just one of those people.

MODELLING AND INHERITANCE

In many families, the idea that cancer is passed down by genetics is a scary thing.

I remember soon after my mom died, one of my cousins approached me and my sisters to see if we should all just get radical mastectomies. Both of our moms had by then died of cancer—this was our chance to end the legacy.

I was only twenty-five years old. My sisters were twenty-three and twenty-one. So here we were with no children yet, our whole lives ahead of us, and yet we were discussing whether it would be the best thing to just go and have our breasts removed.

None of us wanted to. At the time, I figured that it wasn't a good idea because I had heard that the odds were slim that the procedure removed all of the breast tissue anyway, and that you could still get the cancer after all. This didn't seem like good enough odds to me.

This kind of fear is a reality when we look to our genes to explain disease. The idea that we are physically hard-wired for the disease carries with it a sense of inevitability.

But when I look at me and my mom, I wonder what else is passed down from parent to child. I wanted so much to be like her. I wanted to think like her, dress like her, have friends like her, and laugh like her. I wanted to have a great husband, a bunch of kids, and the whole package.

So what else did I get from her? I definitely got her genes. But what else was included in my inheritance?

OUR PRIMARY EDUCATION

Up until a certain age, we learn everything there is to know from our parents. We learn their beliefs, their thought processes, and their ideals. We learn whether or not the world is a safe place. We learn how to celebrate and how to handle stress. We learn how to interact in marriage, on the street, and with children. We learn views on politics, religion, education, work ethic, and social mores.

Is it a formal education? No. It is mostly subliminal. The education is all of the things that we hear around the kitchen table—small talk, stuff that you don't even realize that you are listening to or recording somewhere in your being. As children, we simply observe our surroundings and take them for what they are. We learn that women do "this," men do "this," and dogs do "that." We learn that "this" is acceptable and "that" is not. It's quite simple.

And for all intents and purposes, these things are passed down to us from our parents. We inherit them. They are something that we can carry with us for the rest of our lives and then pass on to our children.

When Disease is Part of the Inheritance

So what if some of our parents' habits and beliefs aren't particularly healthy? What if there are aspects of their personalities and thoughts that lead to disease? If we then imitate those parts of them, it is possible that we might also "inherit" their diseases.

For example, let's say that you are a man who suffers from ulcers. It is common knowledge that ulcers are linked with stress—particularly worry. Where would you have learned this response to stress? Most likely, you learned it from your mother or father.

So let's say that, as a child, you watched your dad come home each day after work completely stressed out. What if he worried constantly about his job security, whether he was doing a good enough job, whether his clients were happy with his work, the state of the economy, and so on?

Without knowing it, you would pick up many things over time. You would pick up the habit of bringing the stresses of work home with you. You might become overly concerned with the opinions of others. You might pick up the belief that you can't ever feel too safe—the rug could be pulled out at any time.

So, if both you and your dad suffered from ulcers, was it a genetic link or was it due to other personality traits and beliefs that you shared?

What if your dad was a real go-getter, Type A personality? Let's say he was aggressive in business, in play, and at home. Everything got done and it got done right. He was driven, successful, and your hero.

These impressions would become your worldview. From a young age, you would learn certain truths—you've got to work hard to get ahead, it's a dog-eat-dog world out there, there's no time to be patient, you've got to be the best, etc.

If your dad has a heart attack, and then you grow up and have a heart attack too, was it a genetic predisposition? Perhaps. But perhaps there is more to it than that.

THE FAMILY LEGACY OF BREAST CANCER

And then there's breast cancer.

Since breast cancer is passed down the maternal line, from mother to daughter, we must ask ourselves, "What else specifically is passed down from mother to daughter?"

The number one thing that we learn from our mothers is how to be a woman. We learn what it means to be a woman, what our role in the family is, what our role in marriage is, and what our role in the community is. We learn how to care for ourselves (or how not to). We learn our importance, our place, and how much we are to expect out of life.

It's not intentional and most of it is never said out loud. But a daughter is always watching her mother—how she moves, how she interacts with people, how she talks. She learns what rights she has in marriage, as a mother, as a woman in society. The modelling impact is massive.

And if the "breast cancer personality" is part of the package, what will the girl imitate? Being selfless. Always being aware of everyone else's needs. Never appearing unhappy. Swallowing her words to avoid making waves. Taking other people's opinions to heart. Never saying "no" to anyone.

And on the surface, this sounds great, altruistic even. But with those things also come the exhaustion, the inner turmoil, and the depression that comes from never living your own life. Unfortunately, even this will seem normal to her because she will have watched her mom be the same way.

For years, oncologists have been noticing these kinds of patterns in women who get breast cancer. They see women who are people-pleasers—women who are overly concerned with other people's needs, opinions, and expectations. They are people who don't share their feelings if they think it might bother someone, and they tend to put everyone else's needs ahead of their own.

There is a high likelihood of young women imitating their mothers because being loved like these women are loved is something that we all want. And so, there is every reason in the world to mimic everything that their mothers ever did, felt, or believed.

So, if we mimic all of these selfless qualities of our moms and end up with the same disease as them, was it strictly genetic programming? Or was there more going on?

Chapter Seven

God on Top

At the Gate of the Year

I said to the man who stood at the gate of year,
"Give me a light that I may tread safely into the unknown."
And he replied, "Go out into the Darkness and put
your hand into the hand of God.
That shall be to you better than light and safer than a known way."

M. L. Haskins

"So, what does it mean that God has to be on the top of my pecking order?" I asked. "How does that work?"

Jim took a moment to consider. "Well, you understand why 'Self' has to be above everyone else—you have to be running the ship. But where do you get your orders from? Does this just mean that you get to do whatever you want? That doesn't seem very enlightened, does it?

"Inside of each of us is a voice that gives us wisdom. It doesn't want, need, or desire anything. It just tells us the truth. It answers our questions whether we want to hear the answers or not. This is what I call the voice of God."

Using the Term "God"

I'd like to break from the story for a moment to discuss an important question: What is God?

This is a very difficult—some would even say impossible—question to answer. Wars have taken place over this topic all over the world for as long as humans have believed that some kind of higher power exists.

Because of this, it can be difficult to discuss God in a way that will make everyone comfortable. But it is an absolutely necessary topic in the path to health and happiness.

We all have a slightly different idea of what God is. To some, God is an external force that guides us from way out there somewhere. To some, God resides inside of us, perhaps in our heart. God is that divine spark within each of us.

To some, God is eternal energy. This energy is what we are made of. It is the energy that cannot be created or destroyed. This energy could be described as light—the building blocks of every atom in our bodies.

To some, God is described as the eternal void. It is the void that all things come from and are born out of. It is not nothingness. It is intentional void, beyond our comprehension.

Then there are some who don't believe in any kind of God per se, but rather some kind of natural and universal power or set of laws that in some way governs the universe. And between and beyond all of these differing interpretations of God are countless other variations.

I feel that God is all of these things—and not exactly any one of them. They all hit on some element of truth. But none can be perfectly definitive.

Describing God is like the story about the blind men standing around an elephant. The man holding onto the trunk declares, "Elephants are long like a snake." The second man standing by the tusk says, "Elephants are hard and smooth like stone." The third man standing by the leg says, "Elephants are tall and round like trees." And so on.

The point is that elephants are some combination of all of these men's experiences. I believe it is the same with God.

God is called by many names. For the purposes of this book, I am going to use the term "God." (In day-to-day life, I tend to use "the Big Guy." But that's not quite suitable here.)

It is just a word. It is simply a placeholder to represent a much greater entity or force than we human folk could ever imagine. So, as we continue the story, please substitute whatever term brings you the most peace—whatever word gives you the greatest ability to trust and have faith in yourself and the process.

HOW DO I HEAR THE RIGHT VOICE?

"So how do I tell what God is saying?" I asked Jim. "It's easy to figure out what my family and friends want and need. And I am learning to figure out what I want. But how do I know what God wants?"

"I suppose that it's different for everyone. But in my experience, God speaks to us through our hearts. This is where our Truth resides."

"So, I go by my feelings? I do what I feel like?"

"Not really. It is actually simpler than that. There are two primary emotions—happy and sad. All other emotions are secondary. When you are faced with any kind of decision, your heart will immediately register one of these two emotions—happy or sad. 'Happy' feels like your heart lifting—the idea excites you. 'Sad' feels heavy—you probably don't want to do it."

I thought about this "happy vs. sad" idea. I had had this experience a thousand times before. The phone would ring and it would be someone asking if you would like to do something. The moment they ask, your heart gives a little lift or a little drop. I knew what that was like.

For example, let's say someone calls and wants you to take squares to the bake sale at the school. As soon as they ask, your heart immediately falls. You don't have time for this. You are already maxxed out. But everyone's parents are contributing. It's the least you could do for the fundraiser. You don't want to be the one who says no. So you say, "Sure. How many would you like me to bring?"

But inevitably, the whole process becomes a mess. The oven doesn't work right on that day, or you don't have the necessary ingredients, or your car won't start on your way to the school and you end up getting there late for the bake sale after all. You think, "Man, I should have just said no right up front."

Or alternatively, your girlfriend calls and invites you to go away for a girls' weekend. Let's say that your heart immediately skips a beat. "Oh, yes!" it is saying. But then reality kicks in. Your daughter is in a soccer tournament this weekend and you said that you would go to the in-laws' for lunch on Sunday. And there is just so much laundry and the house is a mess. You really couldn't go away. So you sadly say, "I'd really like to, but I just can't swing it."

Then you take your daughter to her soccer tournament, but you're unable to enjoy it, and you resent the hell out of your in-laws for making you have lunch at their place on Sunday. The house doesn't get any cleaner and the laundry doesn't get done because you were so upset that you didn't go away for the weekend. Instead you devoured a bag of chocolate chip cookies and didn't have the heart to bother with the housework.

Yes, this phenomenon was familiar to me. However, I seldom listened to my heart. Oh, I listened to it when it agreed with what everyone else wanted to do anyway. But would I listen to my heart if it meant making waves? Would I listen if I would be risking making someone else disappointed, upset, or angry with me? Would I risk the confrontation?

Plus, people want explanations when you don't give them the answer that they want. They say things like, "Why would you do something like that?" or "Why wouldn't you do something like that?"

We have to have good reasons for disappointing someone. We can't just say, "Oh, I just don't feel like it," or "It doesn't feel right in my heart," or "God doesn't think I should do that right now." Most people just don't take these reasons very well.

But this is the leap of faith. This is where you start listening to that little voice instead of the expectations of other people. This is where you stop and consult your "inner guide" before making the decision.

When I was learning to do this, a friend told me to put a sign above my telephone. It said, "Let me think about it. I'll call you later." This sign saved my life. My knee-jerk response had been to just say yes to everything. But then I would look at my little piece of paper, and I could tell them that I'd call them back and then really sit down and think about what the best path was.

WHAT DOES GOD FEEL LIKE TO YOU?

Each of us feels this differently. For centuries, poets, prophets, and philosophers have been trying to define, describe, and encapsulate what the essence of God really is.

But all you need to know is what it feels like to you. You need a reference point—something that you can think about that invokes that certain, special feeling that feels like God to you. It is possible that the English language can't properly or completely convey what that is, and that's okay. As long as you can describe or feel it for yourself, then you'll have that touchstone.

Here's what it is for me.

There is something inside of each of us that understands that we are more than just the flesh and blood that everyone else sees. We know that there is something else. Some might call it a divine spark. Some might call it the Holy Spirit.

We feel it when we hear a piece of music that makes the hair on our arms stand on end. We feel it when we walk in a warm rain and we tip our faces up to feel it and time stands still for a moment. We feel it when we check on our kids in their beds at night and no matter how hard the day was, all is right with the world just staring at those innocent, sleeping faces.

This is that presence. It is the life force that animates this bunch of skin and bones. It is that something that sets us apart from the machines. It is that something that makes us intrinsically human.

It is our connection to something else. Something bigger. Something that transcends all of the problems and stresses of our day-to-day life.

This is what God is to me.

So, how does this work in our pecking order?

This is where we trust our instincts, our hunches—those little nig-glings that chew away at us until we finally do something about it.

This is where we throw away all logic and simply go with our guts.

We say things like, "I just felt called to do it," or "I felt compelled," or "I just knew it was the right thing to do."

We have all had experiences with this. It is when an idea pops into our heads to take the family to Algonquin Park even though we have never been there and we know nothing about it. But we follow our hunch and have the best family vacation ever.

Or, alternately, we have a bad feeling about something—perhaps about taking the freeway to work. So, we take an alternate route only to find out later that there was a massive multi-car pileup on the freeway that morning.

To apply this to our pecking order, we can take it one step further. When we are making a decision in our lives, we can actually stop for a moment and ask, "What is my heart telling me? What rests easiest with my conscience?"

TRUST IN GOD

Faith is not anti-intellectual. It is an act of man that reaches
beyond the limits of our five senses.
Billy Graham

Before I started on this journey, I had a very intellectual belief in God. I had studied religions from all over the world. I was raised in a Christian home with my grandpa being an Anglican minister. But living on the inside of a minister's family also gives you the unfortunate view of the politics that go on inside the church. To say that I ended up a little disenchanted with the whole thing would be a bit of an understatement.

But I was always interested in religion. I studied Buddhism, Judaism, Islam, Hinduism, and Native beliefs. I had studied philosophy and Taoism. During university, I was an agnostic—I would believe in God if you could prove it to me.

But as I got older, and definitely after I had kids, I stopped wondering if God existed. I was sure that God existed. I had experienced too many amazing things to believe anything else.

But it was still an intellectual belief. That God existed was the only logical explanation for things that I had witnessed and experienced. There was no other way that I could have gone through and survived the things that I had without some greater force putting the pieces in place for me.

But this journey changed everything.

This process forced me to have a relationship with God. No more logic. No more reasonable explanations. I had to learn to trust that Divine part of myself. No more head—just heart.

When you are looking for guidance in your life (especially in life and death situations), all the intellectual ideas about God don't serve you one bit. If you don't have a strong habit of listening for and trusting that guidance, if you haven't developed that "muscle" inside of yourself, then you have nothing to help you.

This was huge for me because it meant that I had to start guiding my life without my mind. I had to trust something that I couldn't see. And I had to make decisions based on that guidance.

Chapter Eight

The Battle between the Head and Heart

The heart has its reasons that reason knows not of.

Pascal

I went to Jim's about once a week. Each week, he would do various things with me. But mostly we would talk. The lump seemed to be shrinking a bit—enough to keep me motivated. But I was getting really tired.

I wouldn't say that I was more tired than I had ever been. Maybe I was just noticing it for the first time now. I normally never would have slowed down long enough to notice how I was feeling. And now that I did, I realized that I was *really* tired all of the time.

"Jim, why am I *so* tired?"

"It is this battle between your head and your heart."

"What battle?"

"You know—your heart says no, but your head says yes. Then your heart says, 'But I don't want to.' And then your head says, 'Look! It is the right thing to do. It is what a good mother/wife/friend/daughter/ employee/boss would do! Why are you being so selfish? What is wrong with you? Why would you make a decision like that?'

"And the heart says, 'Because I don't want to.'"

It was true. My mind was always thinking, discussing, arguing, or wrestling with something. It never quieted down. The interesting thing is that the discussions always seemed to be with me. Or my mind would put someone else in the opponent's chair like Wayne or his parents or my dad or my boss or the neighbours or whoever. I couldn't count the endless discussions I had in my head every hour of every day. And I know for sure that most of them weren't productive.

"If you want to get better," Jim continued, "you have to stop your mind—just turn it off. Otherwise, you don't have a chance. I can't stress enough to you how important this is."

"I can't turn off my mind. That's like asking a marathon runner to stop running. I can't even begin to imagine what it would be like to turn off my mind!"

When I imagined turning off my mind, it felt like the entire world would just come to a screeching halt. Everything that I had planned for my kids, my family, and myself would just end. The plans would never come to fruition. Not to mention all of the daily problems and challenges that had to be dealt with. How could anyone function with their mind turned off?

Unfortunately, trying to think my way out of this one was impossible. There is no amount of thinking that will help you stop thinking. It just doesn't work.

"So how do I do it?"

"Do what?"

"Turn off my mind."

"End the battle."

"How do I do that?"

"Start honouring your pecking order. If God is on top and he speaks through your heart, then live according to your heart. Don't let your brain bully your heart out of its desires. Just say no. This is the only way to end the battle. Take all of the power away from the mind. Empower the heart."

This seemed simple enough. I could do that. But what would I say to people? I could no longer give them explanations for why I was or wasn't doing something. But maybe that wasn't so important. It wasn't really any of their business anyway. And again, I was sick. People give you a lot more space to do weird things when you have breast lumps.

"But then what do I do when I actually have to make a decision about something? Don't I need my mind at all in the process?"

THE BRAIN CAN'T MAKE DECISIONS

"What you have to realize is that the brain is actually incapable of making decisions. Decision making is not its job. No matter how hard you think about something, you will not be able to make a decision. In fact, the smarter you are, the more impossible it is for the head to make any decisions at all."

"What?"

"Think about it. When you use your mind to analyze a situation in order to make a decision, the more intelligent you are, the more you can see both sides of the situation. It is only a small mind that can only see one side and therefore the conclusion is obvious. But if the mind can see the pros and cons of both sides, how can it make a decision? If it truly understands both sides of the situation, it will drop into 'analysis paralysis.' It is utterly incapable of making the decision."

"So then, what happens? We do make decisions eventually."

"We generally will have had a preference from the start. There will have been a feeling—a gut instinct. Let's call it 'A.' After this gut feeling, one of two things will happen. One, we listen to our heart because all of the analysis and everyone we talk to agrees that 'A' is the right choice.

"Or two, the analysis and our friends think that 'B' is the right answer. But we find ourselves endlessly arguing for 'A.' Eventually, we might choose 'B' to please our friends, but we regret it. Or we choose 'A' after all. We don't understand why, but we choose 'A.'

"The funny thing is that we could've saved ourselves the trouble and hassle and simply listened to our heart in the first place."

I think I understood this. You can often tell when this battle is going on in someone else. You know it because when you see them, they start to tell you about a decision that they have made. Then they spend the next hour explaining to you why they did it that way. You are sitting there wondering why they are going into this huge explanation. You don't even have an opinion on their decision. It means nothing to you. But they will be in there in spades explaining to you every detail of their reasoning.

The truth is that they are not really talking to you. You are just witnessing the battle between their head and their heart.

"So, if it is the heart's job to make decisions, then what is the mind's job?"

"The mind manifests the decision. It makes the plan. It figures out how to do it. It's that simple."

Well, this just opened up a huge can of worms for me. I was devastated by how many times during the day I didn't listen to my heart—practically never. I really never even paid attention before. I tended to be just scanning the crowd for answers more than asking myself what I thought.

Before I would ask my heart what was right, I would think, "What would my kids want? What would Wayne want? What would 'whoever else' want?"

That's when the battle within me would start. If I imagined that they wanted something different from what my heart wanted, then I would end up with an argument inside of me. My mind would start coming up with reasons for doing it in a way that would please the others. My heart would say, "But, but, but," and the battle would wage on endlessly.

It's amazing how often we use our brainpower and its unlimited imagination to beat our heart into submission. It just isn't right.

Imagine this scenario: Let's say that you have been wanting to find a passion in your life. You have spent your life up until now catering to everyone else and you want to have time for you. You don't really have time because you have a young family to take care of. But you are exhausted and depressed, and you don't want to go down this road any longer.

But you don't know what you want to do. It's been so long since it mattered what fired you up, you just don't know any more.

And so you ask the Universe. You pray. You set the intention that you want to have some fun and be passionate about something.

And one day a small voice inside says, "I'd like to play the piano."

Let's listen to the possible dialogue that ensues between the head and heart:

Heart: I'd like to play the piano.

Head: You can't play the piano.

Heart: But I'd like to try.

Head: We can't afford it.

Heart: We can afford lessons for the kids.

Head: It's important for their growth and well-roundedness. It's just frivolous for you.

Heart: I think that I'd enjoy playing the piano.

Head: When are you going to do this? You don't have time to get done what needs to get done now! Between making supper for the family and running the kids to their events, when would you have time? You can't expect them to feed themselves just so you can go off and spend time on something unimportant.

Heart: I think that it would be good for me.

Head: Would you really practice? When is that going to happen? It's a waste of time and money if you don't practice. And where would you use it anyway? It's not like you're going to be a concert pianist...

Are we cruel or what? The heart cannot justify its decision. It is simply speaking the desires of the soul. It can't match the endless arguments that the mind can come up with.

The truth is that we will never know why we wanted to play the piano until we do it. Maybe it is the teacher who will change our world. Perhaps the process of learning enlivens something inside of us that we didn't know was there. Maybe our daily practice becomes guaranteed "me time." Maybe we just love the sound of Bach and it opens up something beautiful and alive inside of us. Who knows? But we won't know until we try.

SHUTTING OFF THE MIND

But shutting off the mind isn't easy. We have been training our minds to make decisions since our first day of kindergarten when we were five years old. We were graded on our mind's abilities to learn and make the right decisions for the next twelve years or more. This concept is embedded in our beings.

I had an honours degree in mathematics. My mind was very accustomed to making many decisions and solving many difficult problems.

But that was just mathematics. We aren't talking about deriving statistical formulae, figuring out how much your loan payment will be, or what your car's fuel economy is. These are all simple calculations. And do you know why they're simple? Because we have all of the information in front of us. All our brain has to do is the math.

OVERSIMPLIFYING LIFE

But life isn't that simple. There are all kinds of variables out there that our brains don't know about. In fact, there are so many variables in the real world that our brains have to ignore most of them just to stay sane.

To do this, our brains simply take in what they understand and disregard the rest. So when a situation arises, our brain takes all of the information that it can understand, matches that up with all of the rules and regulations that it knows of, and judges which solution is the most logical.

It's very simple and very logical. But unfortunately, it is often totally wrong.

It's like looking into your neighbors' lives, deciding what is wrong with them, and then deciding what is wrong with it, and then deciding what the best path is for them. In order to do this, we would look at the parts of their lives that we can see and understand. We might consider their financial situation, what jobs they hold, what we know about their wayward children, how well they take care of their property, and any other gossip that we have heard.

In reality, these pieces of information would barely scratch the surface of what is really going on. But in order for our brains to feel like they have come up with a clever solution, we must ignore things like their upbringings, their depression, their personal losses, their health problems, their panic attacks, the relationships between their kids, their marital problems, their religious beliefs, and the thousands of other aspects of their lives that are affecting them at any given moment.

Simplifying is neater but not all that applicable to real life. In fact, scientists are finding the same thing.

For man-made objects, such as a car, the old science that we learned in school works really well. We know all of the moving parts. We understand all of the forces that are having an effect on them. We know all of the chemicals that might have a reaction. Why do we know all of this? Because we created the car ourselves.

In cases like this, science can do amazing things.

But over the years, many scientists have realized that their old science just doesn't cut it when trying to understand anything that we didn't build. Think of the weather. Our science can't predict tsunamis. It can't do anything about hurricanes, drought, excessive precipitation, tornadoes, or any other weather.

We find the same thing happening in medicine. When you have been in a car accident and your leg has been seriously damaged, the doctors understand all of the parts that they are dealing with. They understand how the accident happened and the extent of the injuries. They understand how the body heals itself when all the parts are placed back together just so. They understand how to keep the body out of shock so that the patient will survive the surgery.

But when they're dealing with diseases like cancer, headaches, asthma, fibromyalgia, or the common cold, the problem is that they just don't have all of the pieces. Just looking at the physical body isn't giving them enough information to help. And so, they do what they can to ease the pain and hope for a cure.

But doctors like Carl Simonton have long been noticing other "pieces" that are important in healing cancer—like the fact that many people who get cancer tend to be people-pleasers. Bernie Siegel noticed that many of his cancer patients who got better had unique personalities and weren't afraid of standing out in the crowd. Deepak Chopra observed phenomenal inner shifts in people just before their cancer literally disappeared.

These are pieces of the puzzle that cannot be ignored. And so, scientists are now looking for clues in other places. They are starting to look into the mind. They are looking at emotions. They are looking at lifestyles, relationships, and spirituality. These are things that the mind cannot understand. It isn't simple enough. But this is the new research. This is the new frontier. It is out of the simplistic ideas of the left brain and delving into the more intuitive side of the right.

Simple just isn't cutting it anymore.

Programming and Other People's Ideas

Another reason to shut off our minds is that this is where we store all of our past programming. This is where we keep our parents' ideas, prejudices, ideals, beliefs, cultural mores, and opinions. This is where we store what our teachers expected and thought of us. This is where we know what church and society taught us. This is the judge and jury that we carry with us every day.

But we don't want old programming to dictate what our lives are like right now. There might have been a certain way that our parents chose to live. But now, we want to make decisions that are relevant today. Maybe there was a certain way that society thought about things in the past. But today might require different solutions.

Then we have to add the people in the present. It is in our minds that we have all kinds of discussions with the people in our lives right now.

It might be the voice of our spouse: "What will he think if I do that?"

It could be the voice of our children: "Will they still love me and think that I am a good mother if I do this?"

Or what will your friends, neighbours, colleagues, or family think?

And what about the future? Do you have fears about your children lying on their therapist's couch one day talking about how their mother ruined their lives?

These are all fears and concerns that live in our minds. Sometimes, they are worth listening to. Sometimes not. But the mind cannot make this decision either. It can't see within its own maze. It needs the heart to sort through it all and make decisions in the here and now.

Truly Responding to the Present Moment

Shutting off the mind is the only way to respond in the present moment. The mind is good at remembering the past and projecting into the future. But it struggles to respond in the here and now.

To truly respond, you must primarily feel your way. If your brain is doing the job, then you are reacting. You are pulling up old files that hopefully will apply to this situation.

Let's say you need to respond to a difficult situation. Your sixteen-year-old daughter has fallen in with a tough crowd and is getting in trouble at school, and you are very worried.

Are you going to talk to her with your brain? Explain to her all the reasons that she doesn't want to be doing what she's doing?

We all know that this doesn't work. And do you know why this doesn't work? Because she has already heard everything that you are going to tell her. She has already received that programming from you, her school, and society. The fact is that she is choosing to override it. This is what is interesting to you. This is what you care about.

Going "head to head" is not the answer here. You are not going to reach your daughter. In fact it might escalate to a place that you definitely didn't want to go.

You must shut off the brain *completely* and dive 100 percent into the heart. This is the only way.

When you do this, there is a chance that she will also turn off the mind and go into the heart. As long as the mind stays shut off, you both are in a safe place to share honestly and openly. Now you have a chance at a real relationship and a real connection. This is your goal. But as long as the mind is engaged and judging and fearing and coming up with solutions, it's unlikely that you are going to be able to help at all.

Exhaustion

Exhaustion is the result of not shutting off the mind and allowing the battle to go on and on.

Monkey mind is a Buddhist term for a mind that is unsettled, restless, confused, indecisive, and/or uncontrollable. This is the mind that exhausts us to our very core. It is the mind that never stops planning and wondering and worrying and regretting and stressing and thinking.

It never stops. It doesn't let us sleep. It doesn't let us focus. It doesn't let us live.

We feel like we are doing a lot because our minds are so active. But when the monkey mind is going, we are like the person sitting in a rocking chair rocking away, thinking that they are going somewhere because they are working so hard.

Shutting off our minds is like taming this monkey mind. We learn how to shut it off when needed and how to take it out when needed.

This allows us to find stillness. We can find our centre. It gives us a chance to rest and to heal.

CHAPTER NINE

RELATIONSHIPS WITH OTHERS

It is easy in the world to live after the world's opinion;
it is easy in solitude to live after your own;
but the great man is he who in the midst of the crowd
keeps with perfect sweetness
the independence of solitude.
Ralph Waldo Emerson

When I was first dealing with my lumps, I felt like I needed to distance myself from many people. I didn't want to talk about what I was going through. I didn't understand the path myself and so I couldn't really explain it to anyone else.

I needed to explore this new way of seeing and interacting with the world around me without anyone's outside influence. There were very few people that I could talk to about this, which was probably good because one of the tendencies that I was trying to overcome was being overly dependent on what other people thought.

I even had to put a little space between me and my sisters. They had always been very close and supportive. But they were raised in the same home that I was and had all of the same training and programming that I was desperately trying to sort through and undo. Their opinions and concerns about my process were not going to help me here. They didn't understand it and their well-intended arguments would often weaken my resolve. That was not what I needed.

The truth was that I didn't know where the path was heading. I seemed to be continually stepping into the abyss, not knowing what was coming next. So, most of the time, I didn't really have anything interesting to share anyway. I just plodded on asking for guidance and trying to hear the answer.

It was only after the lumps were gone that I shared all of the truths that I had found along the way.

Taking a Little Distance

This need to create some distance isn't a bad thing, nor is it permanent.

But if we are ever to figure out what *we* really think and feel about things, at some point, we must step back from our relationships and stand alone. Our relationships are a big part of our lives. But up until this point, they might not have been the healthiest for us.

The people around us are woven into who we are in a very intimate way. And in this process of finding our personal paths and listening to the intelligence within us, giving ourselves a bit of space is absolutely necessary so that we can reformulate these relationships in a new and healthy way.

If a relationship is abusive or dysfunctional, it is obvious that it needs to be given some real space. These might be relationships that we have allowed because of circumstances, work, or just politeness. It is usually easy to allow some distance in these relationships, especially if we are dealing with a serious disease.

The harder ones to give some space are those that aren't particularly bad or obviously dysfunctional. But they still might be unhealthy. It might be a loving spouse, caring siblings, well-meaning friends, or parents that we need to step back from for a time.

We are often so interwoven with these people that we can't tell where we end and they start. We just don't know what are our own ideas and dreams and what are theirs. We don't have to physically leave them—just psychically when we are making decisions and trying to listen to our own hearts.

The problem is that we are often dependent on our loved ones to help us to make decisions. When we want to do something, we might use them as a sounding board and throw some new ideas at them. But often, we are actually trying to convince them that what we want to do is okay or that our ideas are valid. We are depending on them to validate our ideas instead of just believing in them ourselves.

If we ever want to be able to trust our own decision-making process, using our pecking order to stay in line with our truth, then getting rid of this crutch is absolutely necessary.

Now, there might be times when the little voice says to call a certain person for advice. And maybe the discussion that you have with that person will be just what you needed to hear at that time. Then that's fine too. You don't want to become a lone wolf, cutting yourself off from everyone around you. But you need to be able to tell the difference between asking someone for advice in order to make a decision and pretending to have a discussion with someone when you're actually trying to convince them that the decision that you want to make is okay.

THE INABILITY TO BE HONEST WITH OTHERS

Many people who get cancer have an extremely difficult time being honest with others. It isn't that we are overtly lying or trying to deceive anyone. We do it to make it easier on them. We do it so that people will think well of us.

We don't want to hurt anyone's feelings. We don't want to disappoint anyone. We don't want to give anyone reason to be afraid or worried about us. We want to live up to everyone's expectations of us. We want to be approved of. We want to be loved.

And so, we aren't completely honest about how we feel. It isn't that we're being manipulative because we are unconsciously lying to ourselves too. If we truthfully feel a certain way about something and that flies in the face of what our loved ones could accept, we just lie to ourselves about it. So we create a different reality where we think and feel in the way that is expected and then share this new reality with everyone around us. We don't do this consciously. We just can't honour our inner truth. And the more we can convince everyone else that our new reality is real, the more we can convince ourselves.

It's a different kind of lying. But it is a lie, nonetheless.

I remember when my mom was really sick at the end. The bone cancer had eaten away much of her skull. She was on so much morphine that she could barely function.

I remember that people would call to say that they wanted to come over to visit. The neat thing was that this was the first time in her life when she felt she had the right to be honest with them. If she didn't feel like it, she would just say no. No explanation. No justification. She would just say that she wasn't up to it that day. I remember her saying how great that felt—to have the right to say no without any good explanation and without feeling bad that she had disappointed someone.

But then a few days later, she would be feeling a little better. (She wasn't ever feeling good anymore. Every day was just a different degree of awful. But some days she didn't feel completely terrible.) And again, people would call to come over.

Sometimes she really wanted the company, but sometimes she just didn't feel like it. Nevertheless, if she was feeling good at all, she would always falter when it came to honouring that feeling of wanting to be alone. She would hem and haw and wince and finally say, "Oh, okay. Yeah, sure. Come on over around three." Then she would get off the phone and admit that she just didn't really feel like company. My dad would say, "Well, why didn't you say that when they were on the phone? I am going to call them back and tell them to come another day." And my mom would stop him saying, "No, just leave it. It will be fine. I will be fine. Just leave it alone."

And then she would go and sit on the couch kind of quiet and resigned. She just never wanted to cause problems.

But no matter how you put it, when they asked her whether she wanted them to come visit, she was lying when she said yes. And the funny thing is that whether they came or not probably wouldn't have affected those people's lives very much. But now she had to put on a smiling face with the little energy that she had left while deep down berating herself for putting these people's needs above her own truth.

BEING FREE OF THE FEARS OF OTHER PEOPLE

In the movie *Phenomenon*, John Travolta plays a small-town character, George O'Malley, who was hit by a light that came out of the sky. Before that night, George was everyone's friend. During the day, he fixed your car and at night he went to the bar for drinks.

But after the incident, he could suddenly do things that he couldn't before. He could move things with his mind. He could learn new languages in twenty minutes. He could read ten books in an evening. He could find solutions to complex problems that he would have never even thought about before.

The townspeople were really nervous. They didn't like the new person. He was the same guy. But these new abilities were scary to them. Even though he only helped people, they just couldn't handle the change. He was different and that was unnerving. So they started excluding him, talked about him behind his back, and generally just shunned him and left him alone.

And George was really struggling with these changes himself. He couldn't sleep. He didn't know what to do with all of the thoughts in his head. But more importantly, he no longer fit in with the very people that he grew up with—the only community that he had ever known.

But the town's doctor remained one of his allies and knew the struggles he was having. One night in the bar, some of the townspeople were questioning George's intentions and criticizing his new abilities. At this, the doctor flew into a rage.

"Why do you have to tear him down? So you can prove that the world is flat? So you can sleep better tonight?"

It's a funny thing—people's desire to criticize amazing things that happen to other people. As soon as something doesn't fit, it's like we need to prove that it isn't real. Otherwise, we might have to admit that maybe our own worldview is faulty.

I'm not saying to avoid those that you love. But humans have a curious trait—we tend to be very uncomfortable with change. We are terrified of not knowing what is coming next. And though we don't understand everything in our world, we like to think that we do, and that belief, though faulty, makes us feel safe—at least on the surface.

We just need to learn to think for ourselves. A healthy distance might be needed in order to do that.

Chapter Ten

Healing Paths

The natural healing force within each of us is the greatest force in getting well.
Hippocrates

As the weeks went on, the lump went through many changes. It split into two lumps at one point. One of them was reabsorbed into my body. The second one was a little smaller than a golf ball. The lump had always been right under the nipple. But one day, I noticed that it was definitely moving. I called Wayne and showed him.

Suddenly, he freaked out. "You have *got* to go and see a doctor! Who knows what that thing is! Please go and see a doctor—for me."

Wayne had a couple of things going on inside. One, he had been with me during the four years that my mom was in treatment and it terrified him to lose me like that.

The second thing had to do with him being a farmer. A couple of times in his life, he and his dad had gone out to the barn to find that one of their prize cows had died during the night. Since the cow had been in perfectly good health the night before, they would have the vet do an autopsy. Inevitably, they would find that she had had a tumour that had burst open, spreading poison throughout the body and causing her death.

This was not what he wanted to have happen to me. He was terrified that one day that tumour was going to burst inside of me and that would be the end.

And now that the lump was moving, things had just gotten too weird for him to handle. He could only go so far with me and my odd and alternative way of handling this lump situation. He was a patient man and he loved me. But he had just reached his limit.

And so I agreed to go to the doctor—for him.

Truthfully, I wasn't afraid of it being a tumour that could poison me. Right from the beginning, I had this strange vision in my mind's eye of a sunny-side-up fried egg inside my breast. The lump was the yolk and the white part was some kind of protective layer behind it. I always envisioned the "egg" slowly moving to the outside of the breast. The protective layer would simply become part of the breast and the "yolk" part— the lump—would just fall off the outside. Where this vision came from was unknown to me. I didn't normally see things like this. But wherever it came from, it brought me great peace.

I did go to the doctor's office. She didn't say much. My normally chatty doctor was actually pretty quiet about the whole thing. She wanted to run a whole battery of tests to learn more about the lump. I thanked her, but I walked out without scheduling the tests.

I had no intention of being tested. Since chemotherapy, radiation, and surgery still didn't feel right for me, I felt that having the tests done would be a waste of the doctor's time.

I had gone to the doctor for my husband, and I know that if he were me, he would have gone for all of the tests. But he wasn't me. That is the point. He didn't have the breast lumps—I did.

And since they hadn't immediately hospitalized me or anything, I would now get back on my own path. I loved him for his concern, but this was about me and trusting my own inner guidance.

MEDICAL VS. ALTERNATIVE

Most people tend to fall into one of two categories: strictly medical or strictly alternative. And generally, never the twain shall meet!

I would have once considered myself "strictly alternative." However, it seemed that there was a greater lesson in store for me when I got pregnant. I had read all the books. I was going to do it all "naturally." I knew how to do the breathing, the visualizations, the right postures—everything! Women have been having babies without science and medicine for thousands of years. And I wasn't going to need them now either.

I soon learned that the other side of that story is that women have been dying in childbirth for all of those thousands of years too. Without medical help, I would have been one of those statistics, and I wouldn't be here writing this book.

The funny thing is that physically there is no reason that I shouldn't have been able to bear the childbirths. (I've got those childbearing hips, if you know what I'm sayin'!) But after twenty-seven hours of painful back labour that wasn't going anywhere, I happily accepted an epidural and a C-section. Then partway through the surgery, all the anaesthetic completely wore off. I was awake and could feel everything! All I can say is thank God for morphine!

That was an important lesson for me about being open to other options. This "strictly alternative" person now had her eyes fully open to some of the benefits of modern medicine.

When dealing with any kind of illness, it is important to consider all options. There is no one perfect way to cure any disease. There is no magic formula that will work for every person every time. At some point, surgery might be the right path for you. At another time, it might be herbs. Another time might call for homeopathy, radiation, acupuncture, chiropractic, chemotherapy, osteopathy, energy medicine, medication, meditation, or something else.

The important thing is that you choose the path that your body is calling for at that time. And no one can tell you what that path is but yourself. Other people can give you ideas. They can give you testimonials. And this advice is important. It is important to listen to the information being presented to you. But in the end, *you* must be the one to choose which path to take.

THE SACRED COWS OF HEALTH CARE

If you start to consider options outside of the norm for your family, you may come up against some opposition, regardless of your background.

If your family is deeply rooted in modern science and Western medicine, they may be outraged that you might consider investigating acupuncture, yoga, or alternative diets. You might hear things like, "I can't believe you are going to just sit back and do nothing! How could you be so selfish and naive?"

If your family is stronger in more Eastern ideas and back-to-the-earth philosophies, they may be mortified if you suddenly decide to opt for chemotherapy. "How could you be so irrational? How could you do something so invasive and aggressive to your body? What is wrong with you? Who convinced you to do this?"

It is often surprising just how adamant and unsupportive loved ones can be when you step outside *their* comfort zone. But remember that what you are doing is defining *your* comfort zone—what makes sense and feels right to you.

Sometimes, the point of the experience may be to argue with them. You will learn from that too. Listening to your family's arguments can be very revealing for you because what they say will echo some of the same arguments you have heard in your own mind, which will help you understand those arguments and where they came from.

Having a Part to Play in Healing

Many people enjoy the blind faith that comes with trusting a certain system. And you will see this in both the medical and the alternative world. Many people like the sense of security that comes with just sitting back, letting the doctor/practitioner make the decisions, and letting the treatment cure their ills. If that doesn't work, the practitioner will recommend another person or treatment and we can still just be passive in the process. But if survival is your goal, this might not be your best plan.

One commonality among spontaneous healers is that they feel they have a part to play in the healing process. This is a radical shift for most people. The idea that we have an active role to play in our own healing forces us out of the passive victim role that so many of us take when we get sick.

The problem is that when we feel like a victim to the disease and assume a passive "fix me" role, this is also what the body hears. And so, our body—this amazing machine that can conjure up precise pharmaceutical prescriptions for just about anything that ails us—simply lies dormant waiting for something out there to fix it.

As soon as you decide that you want to play a part and that you are taking some of the power, the body can get involved too. The body is capable of nothing short of miracles when all systems are engaged.

Maybe you ask your doctor more questions about procedure options. Maybe you feel the need to take up yoga or start taking certain herbs. Maybe you change your diet and start going for a walk every day.

What you do isn't nearly as important as the fact that you do *something*. It is the shift from observing to playing the game that makes all the difference.

THERE IS ONLY SO MUCH THAT THEY CAN DO

There are certain aspects of our lives that only we can change. A doctor or health practitioner can only do so much. If we are chronically depressed because we are unhappy in our marriage, then no amount of medication will ever boost our immunity enough to heal much of anything. We are the only ones who can either do the work to fix our relationship or end the relationship. No one else can do that.

If we have a job that we hate going to and we don't take any action to change that, what can our doctor do to help with our exhaustion, depression, and lack of libido? We are the only ones who can fix this.

These chronic stressors in our lives are contributing to our chronic diseases. The doctors cannot help us get better while these things are going on. It's kind of like putting a bandage on a cut and then lifting it daily and poking at it. The cut won't heal. But that doesn't mean that the bandage wasn't doing its job.

I remember one woman saying that she didn't want to get a lump removed surgically because she didn't know why it got there in the first place. And if she was doing something in her life that had caused it in the first place, what was the point in having it removed just to have it grow again?

If she had had the surgery and the lump grew back, it isn't that the surgery didn't work. It's simply that there were some other pieces that also had to be taken care of for a complete healing. That's where we come in. That's where we take an active role in our own healing.

Chapter Eleven
An Encounter with Death

It is not death that a man should fear; he should fear never beginning to live.
Marcus Aurelius

One night, I was getting ready to go to bed. I had my pyjamas on and was sitting on the side of the bed when the strangest thing came over me. As I sat there, I was suddenly filled with a "knowing" that I was not going to wake up in the morning. This was it. I was going to die in my sleep.

But strangely enough, I wasn't afraid. The only thing that I can compare it to is a story I once heard about a Native American chief who knew that he was going to die. So, he put all of his affairs in order and walked out of the camp to a sacred stone and lay down and died. He just knew. He wasn't afraid. It was simply time.

Well, I didn't know what to do. I didn't want to die. It wasn't time for me. I sat there on the edge of the bed, unsure as to whether or not I should even lie down. I wasn't ready for this. I wasn't feeling the peace that I imagine the Native chief had felt.

But eventually, I laid myself down and I prayed. I prayed and prayed. You know that saying, "There are no atheists in a foxhole"? Well that was me. After I prayed, I cried.

I cried and cried until suddenly my mind quietened and a voice in my head said, "It's up to you—just choose."

My mind started racing. Up to me? Up to me? Choose? Okay. Choose. It's up to me. The answer was obvious. Wasn't it?

But that was when the big shocker came. I didn't know what I wanted. I had to think about it.

I had to think about it! I didn't know what to choose. Here it came down to the final decision and I didn't know whether I wanted to live or die. My rational mind was saying, "You have a great life! Great husband, great kids—what's wrong with you?"

But this other part of me was just quiet, sad, knowing. Maybe I wasn't *really* all that happy. Maybe I wasn't fulfilled. Maybe my life was actually not what I had hoped for. Maybe I didn't believe that it would ever get any better.

I don't know how long I lay there trying to decide. I can't even tell you whether it was my heart or my head that wanted to stay or go. But, eventually, I chose to live. And as soon as I had made the choice, I had this image of a movie flash through my mind. In the movie were all of the things that I still wanted to live for: watching my kids grow up, my family, my friends, everything.

Then I drifted off to sleep.

When I woke up in the morning, I lay in bed not sure what to do. I had no idea what to make of what had happened the night before. It was absolutely shocking to me that in my darkest hour, I had seriously considered slipping out the back door, instead of continuing to live my life.

On the surface, everything was fine. But underneath, there seemed to be a mutiny brewing. Deep down, I was obviously not happy with my life and the choices I was making. Apparently I had to start making some different choices!

About a month later, it happened again. And again, when the time came to make the choice, I still had to think about what I wanted to do. It was shocking. Apparently, I am an expert at fooling myself during my waking hours—a great "mistress of self-deception," as my good friend would say.

It happened three times before the lump was gone.

I don't really know why it stopped happening. The biggest difference that I remember was the answers I gave each time. Right after I was given the choice to live or die, I would lie there and think about why I wanted to stay. The first time, my reason was to be with Wayne and see my kids grow up. The second time, there was a bit of that but there were also things that I wanted to do for me. The last time, I remember simply wanting to live. There were no big plans, ideas, or hopes—I just wanted to live.

The Reality Check

When confronted with the possibility of dying, we often get a shocking reality check. Being in a serious accident, getting a life-threatening diagnosis, or even losing someone close to us can break through our own self-deception, and for the first time, we really start to see our lives clearly.

Much of the time, we are surrounded by shades of grey—untruths told to us by others and by ourselves. We are told that we should act "this way" and that it is right to think "that way" and that everyone is depending on us to "do that."

We believe that if we do "this" then "that" will happen. For example, if raise our children in a certain way, then they will become happy, well-adjusted people. They will never do drugs, drop out of school, or be unhappy.

In marriage, we believe that if we do our best and fulfill the roles set out for us by our families and society, then everything will be "Leave it to Beaver" perfect. But then we find there is distance in the relationship. Maybe we start to disagree more than we agree. Maybe we start taking separate vacations. Maybe someone has an affair. Maybe nothing worked out like we thought it should.

Why didn't it? We followed the rules. What went wrong?

The problem is that all of these rules and roles and expectations aren't exactly true. Just because you have a warm meal ready at the end of the day doesn't ensure a happy husband and a loving marriage. Somewhere along the line, we are led to believe this. But it is only a half truth—not so black and white, but more a shade of grey.

The possibility of dying clears all that away. There is suddenly no time or energy to spend on grey areas. The only reason we bought into these ideas in the first place was to ensure the kind of future that we wanted—comfortable family, successful career, respect from others, etc. But with the diagnosis of a terminal illness, this coveted future appears to be disappearing. Suddenly this future—the future for which we are denying ourselves the present—might not be there after all.

So what we are left with is much more black and white. We are left with what is true to us. It starts to become crystal clear that we are not responsible for other people's happiness—that they have to make that choice themselves. We know that the important career just isn't that important if we don't enjoy it and would rather be doing something else. We know that no matter how clean the house is and how great the food is, if there is something wrong in our marriage, those things aren't going to fix it.

We start to ask ourselves different questions. We no longer ask, "What should I be doing? What would be best for everyone else? What is the ideal solution?"

Instead, we start to really look inside of ourselves and ask, "How do I like to spend my time? Who do I like to spend time with? What is really important to me?"

It is that old question, "How would you live your life if you only had six months to live?" What would you do differently? What would you add? What would you get rid of? What would you enjoy more?

We stop playing the games we once did. We don't suffer the same fools that we once suffered. In many ways life becomes a lot simpler.

DO WE REALLY HAVE A SAY?

The idea that we actually have a say as to whether or not we live or die can be a little hard to swallow. But it is a more common idea than you might think.

Many patients with terminal illness say things like, "I can't die until my daughter has her baby and I know that they are fine," or "There is too much going on at work for me to die." There is a common unconscious belief that we do have some influence on the course of our illness.

As I was writing this chapter, my sister-in-law came home from her aunt's funeral with an interesting story. A few days before she died, she had told her husband that it was time to go. Her husband staunchly told her that she couldn't leave yet because their son wasn't back from his trip to Vietnam. She had to at least stick around until Friday when he would return.

Sure enough, she stuck around until Friday. Her son returned, he plugged his digital camera into the TV, and they all watched the pictures from his trip. After a nice visit, her son and his wife went home, and early the next morning, she passed away.

When my mom was sick, we would all create milestones for her to live for. Both of my sisters and I got married. We planned anniversary parties. We were constantly trying to think of something to tell her about so that she would have something to look forward to.

Were we doing this consciously? Did we really think that we could prolong her life by planning these things? No, and yes.

It wasn't a conscious thing. But somewhere inside of us, we knew that it might make a difference. We didn't know what that difference was. But we were willing to try anything. And my mom held on against all odds. When she was first diagnosed, the doctors told us that she only had six months to live. Throughout the four years of treatment that followed, we were told this many, many times.

My youngest sister was the last of us to get married. When she did, my mom was there in a wheelchair—a shadow of her former vibrant self. Much of her skull had been eaten away by the cancer, and the medication was so strong that she was barely herself. But we wheeled her to the back of the wedding aisle, she stood up and held on to my youngest sister's arm, and the two of them walked down the aisle together.

Two weeks later, Mom died.

Beyond just "holding on" a little while longer, we can even live and heal against all odds, like Morris Goodman, "The Miracle Man." He was in a plane crash that broke his neck and crushed his entire spine, leaving him with severe nerve damage, unable to breathe without mechanical aide, and incapable of eating or drinking or moving any part of his body. They didn't believe that he would live through the night.

But he decided that he was going to walk out of the hospital the following Christmas. And after months of following the promptings of an inner voice to breathe deeply, as well as help from inspirational tapes and physiotherapists, his lungs regenerated, his nervous system healed, and he truly did walk out of the hospital on his own two feet!

We have this ability. We find it difficult to believe when we aren't sick because our minds are being logical. And because our minds are unable to comprehend that it is possible, they convince us that it is impossible. But anyone who is close to death knows the truth. The closer you get to that exit door, the less power the mind has to convince you of anything. You just know the truth. And that's that.

This is the most amazing thing about people who looked cancer in the face and for some reason said no. They made a choice to live completely differently, turned around, and walked away from cancer for the rest of their lives. This is what all of us want to do. But we are going to do it without the cancer.

REDEFINING WHAT IT IS TO LIVE

So why would we ever choose to die? What is so wrong with our lives that we would even consider that choice?

The problem is that we often have an extremely low bar that our lives need to meet in order to be acceptable. We think that all we need is food in our stomachs, clothes on our back, someone in bed beside us, and that is good enough. If we have all of these things, then we have nothing to complain about, right?

Then why is half the population on Prozac? Why is depression almost the norm?

Because we are designed to be more than that. We have to redefine what it means to truly live.

Imagine the concept of really *living*—not just existing.

What if each day wasn't just getting up and eating and working and sleeping? What if every day was truly a new day? What if you really didn't know what was coming around the bend? What if you truly lived each day with the wonder and excitement of a child? Now that would be living!

Living—not just existing or surviving, but being truly alive—is pursuing dreams and feeling passion and excitement for what you are doing. It is being on a journey, whether that journey means sometimes driving ahead or sometimes just enjoying the scenery.

Seems impossible, doesn't it? It seems so far from where we are that it might as well be a movie. How can we have this kind of life when there are bills to pay, kids to raise, and jobs to do? How can it be like that when our parents need us and the kids need braces? But it is possible, and we can make the changes necessary to make it happen.

We were designed to live with passion, fun, and joy. We were designed to follow our dreams—anything less than this and we will not be happy. Anything less and we might find ourselves considering "slipping out the back door" in the dark of the night, not knowing how we let it get to this point.

It is time to make some changes.

CHAPTER TWELVE
CHALLENGES TO CHANGING

Our dilemma is that we hate change and love it at the same
time; what we really want is for things to remain the same
but get better.

Sydney J. Harris

One day, Jim came over to my house. I was having a particularly
bad day. I wasn't having any luck turning off my mind and that
was driving me crazy.

The lump was getting a little smaller and that was encouraging. But I
was getting pretty tired of the whole thing.

"How are we feeling today?" he said as he strode into the room.

"I don't know. I just can't do it. I just can't turn off my mind. It seems
impossible."

"Are you following your heart?"

"I'm trying. But I don't want to upset anyone. And it seems that things
would really change around here if I started being honest all of the time!"

I was worried about how making the changes required would affect
my husband and my marriage. I worried about whether I would still be a
good mother if I catered to my own needs before my children's. I worried
about how often I would actually choose to go to family events if I only
went when I really wanted to.

He just sat there and looked at me for a while. I never knew what
he was doing when he did that. Deep down, I think I knew what he was
doing. But I could never put it into words. Perhaps he was reading my
aura. Maybe he was studying my irises. I don't know. Truthfully, I think
that he was just waiting for guidance.

We sat in silence for a while and then he smiled.

"Katrina, do you know what?"

"What?"

"I love you. And if you change, I will still love you."

I just sat there staring at him.

Then he said, "Do you know what else? Wayne loves you. And if you change, he will still love you. And do you know what else? Aaron loves you. And if you change, he will still love you. And Taylor loves you. And if you change, she will still love you."

He continued to go through my friends and family, telling me how much they loved me and that if I changed, they would still love me.

And then I broke. I just started sobbing. I cried and cried. Maybe I was terrified of changing. What if everything changed? What if everything that I depended on right now changed? Maybe that was just too much for me to imagine. What if I started being honest with people and they didn't love me anymore? I wasn't sure it was worth the risk.

Some great wall of belief was crashing down around me. Perhaps it was the belief that I had to act in a certain way in order for people to love me. Maybe it was the relief that I no longer had to pretend to be something I wasn't just to ensure other people's love. I don't know. But there was something really huge in these very simple statements that he made.

I believed what Jim was saying. But change is a scary concept. And I felt I had a lot to lose.

OUR SACRED COWS

The challenge is that we have been acting in this "other" way for a long time. We have been putting other people's needs and expectations ahead of our own for quite a while now—and with good reason!

Maybe you have been the good mom. You have put the needs and expectations of motherhood far above your own best interests. Why would you do that? Because that is what a "good" mom does. That is what young children need. When children are born, they truly do need you twenty-four hours a day. They depend on you for survival. The fact that you change the diapers when needed and feed them when they are hungry is exactly why the human race has survived this long.

Maybe you have been the good provider. You have kept the job for the sake of the family even though it might not really suit your deepest needs and desires. Maybe you have worked longer hours because it was the only way to maintain the standard of living that you are accustomed to. Why would you do that? Because it's the "right" thing to do. It's what anyone with a decent work ethic would do to contribute to the family.

Maybe you have been caring for aging parents. Why would you do that? Because you love them and they have always been there for you. The least you could do is to care for them in their later years.

These are all important and "right" ways to be. But are they so important that they are worth denying your true desires and needs? Those dreams and desires are inside of you for a reason. What that little voice whispers to you matters. It is your path. It is your honest truth. It wouldn't be there if it weren't important.

But after a lifetime of listening to the expectations of our society, the truth that our inner voice speaks doesn't seem to be an easy thing to integrate into our lives. These are our sacred cows that we are dealing with—marriage, children, work ethic, and family. That we might struggle with them is completely natural.

But our fears are unnecessary. If we change, the lives of those around us will adjust to that change. Our children will still be cared for, just in an honest way that respects our needs too. Our family will still have what they need, but we will have what we need too. Our parents will still be cared for, but we won't be run ragged, unable to rest or have our own lives.

CHANGING WITHOUT CRISIS

Once you have been diagnosed with a serious illness, it is often easier to make big changes in your life. Those around you are often understanding and supportive when you start saying no more often, expressing your feelings, and being more honest. This helps your process. Your crisis snaps them out of their day-to-day reality too. Your having to face mortality causes them to have to acknowledge it also.

But with your intention to skip the cancer, you will be making changes without the crisis. Those around you will still be caught in their day-to-day existence. There is no awareness on their part that anything different is going on with you.

But your awareness has been heightened. You are becoming aware of truths that you haven't been accepting and feelings that you haven't been expressing. Your perception of the world seems to be changing with every step. So, as you start to put your truth in motion, you may encounter some resistance from those around you—your spouse, your kids, your coworkers—anyone for whom you did things in the past that you actually didn't want to be doing.

But that's okay. To simply say your truth kindly and compassionately is generally all it takes to assuage anyone else's fears that you are changing in a way that will exclude them in the future. Those same fears that kept you from changing might be the same fears that others feel when you do change. So a couple of words of explanation generally work wonders, keeping you on track and keeping everyone else supportive.

You Will Have to Give Some Things Up

A change toward honesty often means that there are comforts that you will not be able to continue with.

There is a certain comfort in fitting in by never making waves. It means that you go along with whatever the group does whether you want to or not. This could be at home, at work, at family functions, or anywhere. As much as you might like to speak up and have your opinion heard, there is the risk of disapproval or argument. In the short term, it is easier to just sit quietly and let the others battle it out.

There is a certain comfort in just smiling and not actually confronting someone who has just offended you. How often do we just sit there and allow people to walk all over us without defending ourselves? As uncomfortable as it is to have someone offend us, our fear of actually confronting these people can keep us quiet. We know what it feels like to just be quiet and take it, and we don't know what might happen if we stand up and defend ourselves. So, up until this point, sitting quietly is actually the most comfortable spot for us.

But with the desire to be honest and honour your own path in life, these comfortable and safe roles won't work any longer. We want to have faith that our opinion does count—that standing up for what we want is okay. We need to believe that we can handle whatever confrontation might arise, and that it is worth it.

Things Will Be Different When You Change

It is important to to consider the fact that if your intention is to change your state of being, then things are going to be different. The existence of the pot of soup is different once the heat is turned up. If you want things to be different, then things are going to be different.

This seems quite logical and obvious. But we don't always totally get it.

If the habit of never saying no to anyone is a problem that you must fix, then once you start saying no, your life will be different—but not for the worse. Things will be better, but there will be other challenges that you didn't have before.

It's like losing weight. Let's say that your present state is overweight. You desire to be a healthy weight. Change is required. Eating less is required. Exercising more is required. This seems simple enough. However, you must consider what this really means.

If you desire to be thin for the rest of your life, then that means eating less for the rest of your life. This means not eating dessert every time it is available. This might mean finding new ways of entertaining yourself at your desk at work when you are bored. It also means really learning how to listen to your body's hunger signals.

The same goes for exercise. In order to make the change to exercise more often, you might have to let the house get a little messier. Maybe the dishes will have to stay in the sink sometimes. You might have to always leave work on time. Your daily priorities might really have to change.

We have this idea that we can change certain parts of ourselves with all other things staying equal. Not possible. We are a complete unit. Everything is affected by everything else—mind, body, and spirit. It is these overall changes and their effects that we must consider.

And so, when we start being more honest with others, when we start expressing our emotions more often, when we start standing up for ourselves, things are going to change. Other people will treat us differently. How we treat ourselves will be different.

But it is certainly a good kind of different.

WHAT IF THEY DON'T LIKE THE "NEW" YOU?

There is always the fear that if you change, that your loved ones won't like the new you. What if I change into someone that they don't know or like?

The reality is that you aren't turning into someone else. You are simply taking off the masks that you have been wearing. You are just letting the real you shine again.

It is like going back to an earlier version of yourself.

Oftentimes, when you remember who you were before you got married and got the responsible job, that person is closer to the real you than the person you look at in the mirror each day. That former self is the "you" before you put on the masks that you had to wear to meet the expectations—both yours and those of others—that come with marriage, kids, and growing up in general.

But your loved ones love *you*. The real you. The person under the mask. They can feel it. They know that version of you intimately. When you take the mask off and start being more honest and truthful, your loved ones not only get to play with your inner self, they also get to play with someone who is genuinely happy and joyful to be free.

You are not going to become someone they don't recognize. You are simply going to be the same person on the outside that you are on the inside.

CHAPTER THIRTEEN
LISTENING TO MY HEART

Let me speak to you regarding the things of which you must
most beware. To get angry and shout at times pleases me, for
this will keep up your natural heat; but what displeases me is
your being grieved and taking all matters to heart. For it is this,
as the whole of physic teaches, which destroys our body more
than any other cause.

physician Lorenzo Sassoli,
to a patient in 1402

And so, I started listening to my heart.

When someone asked me something, I would close my eyes
and try to feel what my heart wanted. Sometimes it was hard to
tell. But it got easier each time I did it.

The interesting thing was people's different reactions to my new decision-making process. When the kids would ask to do something, I would
honestly answer them with a simple yes or no. There was no explanation
because it wasn't a mental process that came up with the decision. I was
simply repeating what my heart said.

If my answer was not what they wanted, they would immediately ask
why. To that, I had no real answer, so I would say, "I don't know. It just
doesn't feel right, right now. Maybe tomorrow." The funny thing is that
they seemed to totally understand this and were perfectly happy with
that answer.

My husband had the benefit of coming to many of my sessions with
Jim. So he knew what I was trying to do. He knew the issues that I was
wrestling with. But he still had some challenges living with me. There
are a million assumptions that we make every day in marriage. There are
expectations that we have of each other that we are not even aware of. Bit

by bit, each of these was tested because there were many times that I no longer simply did what was "expected of me."

Most of the time I tried to be gentle with these changes. Usually I had the presence of mind to say things like, "I don't understand why. I just have to follow my heart on this one. I am really sorry." But it wasn't always that smooth.

When I first started being honest with myself about how I was actually feeling about certain things, I would find myself getting hyper-emotional. It was like twenty years of pent-up anger and sadness were suddenly given the right to be expressed. And I didn't want to suppress it. I was finally feeling things!

After spending my whole life pushing down my emotions, it was like the pathways that once let them be expressed had disappeared from lack of use. Even if I wanted to cry or get angry, I wasn't able to.

So, now that I had given myself permission to actually feel these emotions, I didn't want to suppress anything at all. If I was angry, I wanted to feel what that was like. If I was sad, I wanted to cry until there were no tears left. It was like I had spent so much time at the other extreme of not expressing my feelings, that I had to now experience the extreme opposite in order to eventually find the happy medium.

Needless to say, there were days when it was like the floodgates of some crazy, hormonal woman had been unleashed.

During these times, I would simply voice this fact—that my pendulum was swinging a little further on the emotional side these days, and that I was just trying to allow myself to be honest with my feelings.

I wouldn't say that I enjoyed being so highly emotional—being incredibly sad or angry isn't a nice feeling. But those were the days when things started to feel real for the first time. How I felt counted for something. I was actually a part of things—not just an observer whose feelings were irrelevant.

Feedback Mechanisms

Many spontaneous healers demonstrate this ability to allow their emotions to flow honestly and easily. Doctors call it emotional lability (the word "lability" refers to something's ease or tendency to change). There is something important about this ability to accept whatever emotion you are feeling—whether it be "good" or "bad"—and then respond to it.

Why is this so important? Why does listening to our feelings make a difference in our health? The answer comes from understanding how our bodies and minds use our emotions as important feedback to keep everything on track.

In the science world, human beings would be considered complex systems. We have a billion moving parts, and they all have roles to play in maintaining and keeping us healthy. What is interesting about complex systems is that they are self-correcting. If something is amok, a message is sent through the system to make a correction. These messages are sent through feedback mechanisms.

A child's toy car rolling along the ground is a simple system. It is not self-correcting. If it is given a nudge off course, it stays off course. But if a guided missile—a complex system—is pushed off course, it will make adjustments to get back on course. This is very important.

Our bodies are like that. They are also self-correcting. If we have strayed off course, we have feedback mechanisms that will bring us back on track and in line with our body's goals. If the goal of the body is to live, then it will be constantly working towards maintaining that goal.

If the body starts to overheat, we sweat in order to cool off. If the body's glucose levels get too low, we get a grumbling in our stomachs that sends us to the fridge for more fuel. When we touch a hot stove, our nerves send us a message of pain to make us remove our hand from the element.

We also have many feedback loops happening within the body without our awareness. Our cardiovascular, respiratory, lymphatic, reproductive, digestive, and nervous systems are continually maintained through intricate feedback loops that keep all these systems functioning properly. There is no conscious effort on our part—these feedback loops are part of the system's design.

Our emotions are also one of those important feedback mechanisms. But this is one that we have a role to play in. This is one that we are supposed to listen to and do something about.

When we are on the right track, we have "happy feelings" and the corresponding chemicals are released in our bodies that make us feel great. This is positive feedback that tells us, "Do more of whatever you are doing."

Other times, we have "sad feelings." We don't like these feelings, so our body sends us negative feedback that tells us, "Change something. Do something different."

But do we listen? Sometimes. But those of us who have cancer on our horizon likely don't. We might put our sadness down to hormones. Maybe we just blame someone else and just get on with our lives. Or maybe we don't accept that we have the feelings at all and we stop even scanning the system for information. We aren't going to listen to it or do anything about it anyway.

When we suppress and ignore our emotions, it's like covering up the flashing check-engine light in our car. Even though something is wrong, we ignore it and do nothing to fix it. Whatever is wrong gets worse and gets buried inside of us. These things pile up and only get worse, leading to all kinds of physical and mental problems.

Maybe that is why people who express their emotions more freely tend to heal better than those who don't. When expressed and listened to, their emotions help them to get back on track. They make corrective changes in their lives, and their health and happiness improve.

EXPRESSING ANGER

Anger is one of the most common emotions that we repress—especially if cancer is on our horizon. Why? Because it is often an indication of an unhealthy relationship, that a personal boundary has been crossed, that we are letting people walk all over us, and we don't know what to do with that anger except suppress it.

In the movie *Anger Management*, Jack Nicholson's character describes two kinds of angry people: First there's the guy ahead of you in the checkout line yelling and screaming at the poor cashier. Then there's the cashier who takes this kind of abuse from people every day, day in and day out, swallowing her frustration and anger. Then one day, she pops, brings in a gun, and shoots everyone in the place! The customer and cashier are examples of external and internal anger—both needing anger management. People who get cancer tend to have the internal kind.

Now, this may seem a little extreme. But in reality, something like that happens every day. Things happen that get under your skin. One person says "this," someone else says "that," your mother-in-law comments on "this," and your husband expects you to do "that." And you smile. You're polite. You keep the peace. Then one day, your husband says that he's going to be home for supper at six o'clock. You've had a tough day at work, the kids are fighting, and you've scrambled to get supper ready.

But your husband is late. At six-thirty, he rolls in and finds a red-faced crazy woman waiting for him crying, "I've had it! I do everything for you people!" The tears fall, some stomping about happens, and your husband and children stare at you like you've gone stark raving mad!

Where do you think all of this anger and frustration came from? Certainly not simply because supper was late. These feelings have been around since you swallowed that first bit of negative emotion. Every time we swallow our disappointment and anger, it sits there waiting to come out. Imagine what all that anger is doing circulating through our system all this time.

So what do we do when we are angry? Do we express the feeling? Do we sit with it? Do we pour a drink or eat some cookies? What do we do?

Understanding why we are angry is the first step because oftentimes the anger is a sign that a personal boundary has been crossed. And with people-pleasers, this is a very easy thing to have happen because our boundaries are very wishy-washy, if they are there at all.

WHAT ARE BOUNDARIES?

A boundary is the clear line that separates you from other people. It is the understanding that "I end here" and "You start there."

Before we have the "I am" experience, our boundaries with other people tend to be quite blurry. We tend to take on other people's problems and emotions. People tell us their troubles or we observe their troubles and we immediately want to fix them.

The problem is that deep down, we actually think that *we* have to fix it—even if it has nothing to do with us—when in effect, it is the other person's job. It was given to them to fix. It may sound harsh, but we are actually hurting that other person's growth by fixing their problems for them. How are they to grow if we keep rushing in and fixing everything that comes up? This is their life. They need to live it and grow through the challenges given to them.

Now this isn't easy for us because inevitably, we will be surrounded by people who love the fact that we will fix their problems for them and try to make their lives as comfortable as possible. They will have gotten used to the fact that we do this for them. So, it will take a bit of time and love for them to get used to taking care of their own problems.

When our boundaries are not clear, we also take on other people's emotions. If someone else is sad, then we feel sad. If they are angry, we are angry. This is understandable and it can be helpful at times. But most of the time, it is just exhausting and completely unproductive.

I was like this for the first ten years of my marriage. I was home with the kids and I helped Wayne on the farm. So, we spent a lot of time together. For some people, this might be great. But, for someone like me who had poor boundaries, it was an hourly roller coaster that was completely exhausting.

My husband is a passionate person—a true redhead.

So, every time he would come into the house—breakfast, coffee time, lunch, etc.—there would be a new emotion rising. At breakfast he might be happy, and so I was happy. By coffee time, he might be completely frustrated, and so I too was frustrated. By lunch he might be fine again. But by supper, he was angry with his brother for something. Well, between him, my baby, and my two-year-old, I would end up completely emotionally wrought! And I hadn't even considered how *I* felt throughout the day.

But this was not my husband's problem. It was mine. He was just going through his day feeling emotions as they hit him—his emotional lability was intact. It was me absorbing these emotions—thinking that I was supposed to do something with them—that was the problem. I didn't understand the difference between caring about his feelings and taking on his feelings.

So what does it look like to have clear boundaries?

Boundaries are not walls. Walls keep others out and they hide you from the world. Boundaries are like the boundary of a country. It is just a line in the sand. "I live on this side of the line and you live on that side of the line. There are rules within my country, and if someone chooses to come in for a visit, they must abide by those rules."

Perhaps you expect to be treated with respect. Perhaps you expect your time to be valued. Perhaps you expect people to honour your choice when you say yes or no.

So what happens if someone crosses that boundary? Maybe they don't treat you with respect. Maybe they keep harassing you because you didn't give them the answer that they wanted. What happens? You get angry.

Now, many of us people-pleasing folk simply swallow that anger. What we feel just hasn't been important enough to cause a stir. If we are upset, there is no point in making anyone else upset. Maybe if we let this slide, it will just go away. It is just not worth worrying about.

But the reality is that our boundary has been crossed. Anger is the proper response because it gives us the strength to enforce the barrier. Without that anger, we will likely let that person come and "live in our country" even if they are very badly behaved and inconsiderate. This may seem like a nice thing to do, but it isn't doing anyone any good.

It's like having a beautiful big home and your dream is to take care of foster kids, to give them a chance at a safe and loving life. Now imagine that your brother decides that he wants to come and live with you, and he is forever painting on the walls, stealing the food, disrespecting the other kids, and just causing trouble. He is hurting the very goals that you have set out in trying to help those less fortunate. He is harming you and everyone that you are trying to help.

The same goes for your own personal boundaries. When you let people in who don't respect your rules, they are simply wreaking havoc with your emotional and mental life. You will end up spending so much time just trying to recover from the damage that you won't have anything of any value left over for the people who really need and appreciate your help.

And the problem is that it won't be only one person that will be crossing your boundaries and disrespecting your rules. It will be everybody. It will be your spouse, your kids, your neighbours, your family, your boss, clients at work, and people on the street.

In the end, you will feel like no one is safe and there is no one who understands you. You will feel like you can't trust anyone to honour your needs and desires. You will be on red alert all of the time.

So, get angry. You don't have to have a temper tantrum. But allow the anger to surface. Allow yourself to feel it. If someone needs to back off and get out of your space, use that anger to make them do it. If someone has harmed you and they need to be told the rules of your "country," then use that anger to do it.

Once you take the necessary action to address the cause of the anger, the anger will subside. Its job will be over. It will pass. You will then be free to feel whatever emotion is coming next.

Expressing Happiness

Happiness seems like a funny emotion to withhold. We normally think that it is only the negative emotions that we tend to stifle. But for some people, happiness is hard to accept and embrace too.

For many people, it is hard to be happy if other people are sad, especially if they are close to us. This is understandable. There is a certain amount of natural empathy that you will feel for a loved one who is suffering. But that does not mean that you cannot be happy. You don't need to dance and skip around them while they suffer, but inside you can be clear that maybe you are actually having a good day even if you have compassion for your loved one.

I remember when my mom had cancer. If she got up in the morning and she was having a bad day, then so did we. How could I be cheery at work and enjoy the sunshine when I knew that my mom was at home swelled up on morphine, barely able to speak, and fighting for her life? How could I be so callous as to stop and smell the flowers or enjoy a morning coffee? How cold would that be?

Actually it wouldn't be cold at all. It would be healthy. I was once at a seminar where Wayne Dyer said that "you can't feel bad enough to make another person feel better." These words ring in my head often. No matter how bad I felt, it wasn't helping my mom. In fact, I might have even contributed to the guilt that she felt at what her illness was putting us through!

She didn't want me to be unhappy. Probably the best thing that I could have done was to come home from work happy and full of energy. Maybe it could have boosted her spirits somehow.

If I had of known then what I know now, I would have listened to my feelings. I would have allowed myself to be happy and trusted that that was the best thing for everyone. I would have allowed myself to be sad and maybe my mom and I could have had a big cry together.

But I didn't trust my feelings then. I thought I knew better.

Chapter Fourteen
Guidance and Prayer

Whatever you ask for in prayer, believe that you receive it, and you will.
Mark 11:24

I hadn't been telling many people about the lump. For most of the process, I wasn't strong enough to answer the questions about why I wasn't going the medical route. The truth is, I had chosen a way of faith and I didn't have the words or perhaps the confidence to explain that to anyone.

One day, the minister from my in-laws' church came over for a visit. I had a bit of a history with this guy. He was a nice man whom I respected, but we didn't go to his church for several reasons. I wasn't exactly enamoured with organized religion. I had attended church for many years, but always struggled with much of what the ministers said and just couldn't find the spiritual guidance that I was looking for.

But this guy would come over for friendly visits. I suppose that he was trying to bring us back into the flock. But I think that he just liked the conversation. I think he liked to argue with me. I wasn't intimidated by him. My grandfather and my uncle were ministers. I knew that they were just human beings doing the best job they could. So if the reverend wanted to know what I thought about a controversial topic, I would tell him!

On this day, I chose to tell him about my lump. In the course of the discussion, I told him that Jim had been encouraging me to pray. The reverend's eyes just lit up. We had had many discussions about prayer before, mostly about how I didn't like the way they prayed in church. At this point, he said, "So you do believe in prayer!" I said yes. Then he asked me if we could pray together.

Something started to fume inside of me. I didn't want him praying.

I just wasn't into it. But for whatever reason, I said sure. As he started to pray, I could feel familiar walls going up. But instead of letting them go up, I thought to myself, "If you're going to let him pray, you might as well open up to it."

And then something happened. My whole body started to tingle. And the most concentrated tingles were in the lump in my breast. The sensation continued for the entire prayer. We chatted briefly afterwards, but I was freaked out!

After years of arguing about religion with anyone who came along, the last thing I wanted was to have some kind of mystical experience as a direct result of a man of the cloth praying. My ego and all of my bright ideas were definitely taking a hit for this one.

The next day, a friend called. She and I had had a history of arguing about religion as she was a born-again Christian who truly feared for my soul. So telling her about my tingle experience would really open me up in a vulnerable spot. But it felt right to tell her. So I thought, no time like the present to start trusting this heart thing.

So I told her the story about the tingles. True to my expectation and fear, she burst out with, "Katrina, the Lord is chasing you down. You've got to start reading the Bible!" Well, that was enough of that, and I got off the phone.

Later that day, an old friend from university called me. I hadn't heard from him for about a year. At that time, he had been really struggling with relationships, jobs, and drugs. We had talked about him maybe returning to his Seventh-day Adventist roots to get grounded again.

Well, on this day, I chose to tell him about my tingle experience. And what does he come out with? "Katrina, the Lord is chasing you down. You'd better start reading your Bible!" I was freaked out! It was one thing to hear this from a born-again Christian. It was quite another to hear it from my dope-smoking friend from university.

The next day, I had an appointment with Jim and I told him about my tingles. He promptly left the room and got his Bible and said, "You'd better start reading this."

At this, I lost it. That was it! I said, "If one more #$@%#$ person tells me to go and read my Bible, I'm going to lose my mind!"

Jim looked at me smiling and said, "Katrina, if three absolutely unconnected people tell you exactly the same thing within twenty-four hours, do you not think that it is you who is asking for it?"

THE POINT OF PRAYER

I had asked for this answer. I had wanted to know what to do next. This wasn't the answer that I had wanted. But I had asked for it. And it was pretty clear.

Suddenly, this prayer thing started making sense to me.

We have been taught that prayer was just about asking. You pray for help. You pray before bed and count your blessings. You pray for people who are sick.

But that is where it ends. You pray and then you wait and you trust that God heard you. But this is only part of the process.

The next step is listening for guidance. If you ask for help, you should expect that whomever you asked would answer you! Once I realized this, I started hearing responses in the weirdest places. I would be in my car listening to a song on the radio. It would be a song that I had heard a thousand times and suddenly there would be a line that just replayed over and over in my head. And something would click inside of me— aha! I would then know what to do next. It was truly an amazing thing.

The next, and sometimes hardest, step is following the guidance. This is the true leap of faith. This is also the point where you might start questioning your sanity. You start to ask yourself whether the guidance was really God or something else. Should I be listening to voices in my head telling me what to do? Isn't that what crazy people do? This is where you really test whether you are comfortable with your pecking order, and whether you are truly comfortable listening to that voice inside you.

A FUNNY STORY

There was this guy who was sitting on the roof of his house because a huge storm had ripped through and his town was flooded. He sat on that roof and prayed and prayed for help.

Soon, a man on a raft came by and offered for him to climb on. The man said, "No, thank you. I am waiting on the Lord."

Then someone in a motor boat came by and offered to help. The man repeated, "No, thank you. I am waiting on the Lord."

Finally, a helicopter flew overhead and dropped a ladder for him to climb up on. He waved them on. He was waiting on the Lord.

Well, he ended up dying on that rooftop. And as he approached the

Pearly Gates, he saw God and asked him, "Why didn't you save me? I prayed and prayed. What went wrong?"

"I sent you a raft, a motor boat, and a helicopter. What more could I do?"

THE LISTENING

What does the guidance sound like?

I think that it is different for everyone. For me it is a small voice. It's a quiet voice that just sits in the corner of my being and repeats the same thing over and over again. It doesn't argue. It just repeats my truth every time I ask.

Sometimes, the advice would come out of the mouths of people that I wouldn't expect. I would be having a discussion with someone and they would come out with exactly what I needed to hear. We would just be chatting and suddenly their words would just bore into my soul. And often they would be speaking on a topic that they weren't necessarily that knowledgeable about. But on that day, in that moment, they told me exactly what I needed to hear.

Sometimes I would be walking through a bookstore and a book would nearly fall off the shelf at me. Sometimes, the answer came while I was walking through the woods.

For some the answer might come while going for a run or a bike ride. Or maybe playing an instrument or sketching. Sometimes it is in journaling or silent meditation.

In my experience, it doesn't always come in the same way. We have to keep our eyes and ears open to hear wherever and whenever it might come.

This can be a difficult part because this is where you really have to trust whether what you hear is actually your wisest self speaking. What if it is actually one of the other hundred voices in your head? What if it isn't wisdom? What if it just the voice of some person from your past? What if it is fear speaking?

Only you can decide. Only you can hear the difference between old programming coming up and new guidance coming in.

THE ACTING

This is the true leap of faith. This is where the rubber meets the road and you really decide whether you believe in this stuff or not.

The reason it is the leap of faith is because now you are taking what you heard and putting it out into the world. And you have no good explanation to prove to anyone else that what you are about to do makes logical sense. The best you can do is say, "It just feels right." Unfortunately, our society doesn't have a good understanding of following one's intuition, so most people don't trust it.

But this is where I found that life started getting interesting. This is where I would make the decision, stand back, and watch. After years of making calculated, careful decisions, the idea of taking action based on an inner calling that made no logical sense became pretty exciting.

I think that this is when I really started to come alive.

CHAPTER FIFTEEN
BECOMING WHO YOU REALLY ARE

*The search for one's own being, the discovery of the life one needs
to live, can be one of the strongest weapons against disease.*
Lawrence Leshan

I did start reading the Bible every day. After every meal, I would sit down with a cup of tea, the New Testament, a pen, and a journal— and I would read.

There was a time when I read the Bible quite often. But I used to analyze it. That's not what I was doing now. I was looking for guidance— guidance for right now. And so I'd let my mind wander over the pages until things jumped out at me. And jump out they did!

One time, I was reading the parable of the talents. It is a story about a master who goes on a journey and so he entrusts his property to his servants. He gives a number of "talents" to three of his servants, according to their abilities: five to one, two to another, and one to another. While he's gone, the first two use these talents and make more money for their master. But the third one digs a hole and hides his talent to keep it safe.

When the master comes back, he is thrilled with the first two servants. But he is furious with the third. In fact, he even takes away the talent that he had given him and gives it to one of the other servants.

Well, I had read that story before. But on that day, it completely took my breath away. I was that third servant! I had been given talents and had chosen to hide them away. I had been given talents! But because I was choosing to live as someone else's second-in-command, I was not using them.

But I couldn't blame anyone else. It was me who didn't have the courage to use them. I didn't want to cause a stir, although deep down, I probably would have loved to cause a stir—to be the centre of attention for my talents. But that just didn't fit into what I could imagine at that point.

So now that I had buried my talents, was I in jeopardy of having them taken away? Or had they already been taken away? I supposed that it was a moot point because I wasn't using them anyway.

It was time for me to become who I actually was. It was time to unearth those talents and start honing them and using them. No more hiding. No more pretending to be less than I am.

It was time to truly become *me*.

TRULY BECOMING ME

There's a story about a beggar who sat on a little box every day at the side of the road. He never had enough food or drink or lodgings. He just sat there holding out a cup waiting for handouts. Then one day a wise man came along and asked him what was in the box. The beggar shrugged, "I don't know. I never looked." Well, he looked, and lo and behold, it was filled with gold!

We are like this. We have been sitting on a box of gold all this time.

Our true self is right there under the surface. We don't have to develop or find that self. We just need to stop suppressing it.

So what were these talents that I was hiding? At that point, I had no idea. My life was filled with diapers, dishes, and milking cows. And based on how little I was enjoying things at that point, there was no way that they were my talents.

But what were they then? The fact that I didn't know drove me crazy.

Sure, I had always been good at school. I even had an honours degree in mathematics. But what good was that for a stay-at-home mom of toddlers? I had always loved to dance. But I lived in the middle of the country and there was nowhere to do that either. No matter what I came up with as a possible talent, I had a thousand reasons why it was either impossible, impractical, or not really all that interesting anyway.

So, I started asking people what they thought my talents were. They would say that I was a great listener. Of course, to me, this wasn't a talent. Listening was just something I did because I wanted to understand where the other person was coming from. It wasn't a talent. I was just really curious.

Or people would say that I was great at organizing things, and my head for numbers and bringing many complex ideas together was a really unique talent. Again, I had never considered this a talent as much as the root of my regular migraines. The fact that my mind never stopped churning over concepts and ideas and numbers seemed more like a curse to me than a gift.

It took quite a few years before I really found my talents and was able to use them in my life. I found out that I loved to do counselling and that that ability to listen really was an important gift. Combining my love of dance and my organizational abilities, I opened a dance studio primarily for adults where they could learn anything from tango to cha-cha to belly dance. And the fact that I had read thousands of books, had an opinion on everything, and was a pretty decent writer soon turned into a regular column for our local newspaper.

It was interesting that as soon as I followed one talent, another one would appear. And then as that new one became part of my life, another one would pop up.

But during the lump, I didn't know all of this, and I had to settle with just not knowing. I had to trust that I did have talents. I had to trust that my talents were useful even living out on the farm, that other people might be right about the gifts that they saw in me, and that one day I would have the chance to use them. I had to trust that one day things would be different.

Chapter Sixteen
Living in the Real World

At one particularly low point, I went to see Jim. I'd been feeling really down, lost, and alone. It was like there was no one I could turn to, no one who really understood.

I was questioning the very basic assumptions about what is right and wrong in life. I was questioning all of the training that I had ever received—officially and unofficially.

I was reassessing all of my relationships. I was looking at all of the choices that I had ever made. Sometimes it felt like nothing made sense anymore. I was like a boat that had lost her moorings. Sometimes it was all really scary.

Wayne was there supporting me, but he was worried. He was scared that I would have the same fate as my mom. He wanted to trust that I was doing the right thing. But he was struggling with it. I couldn't go to him when I was having doubts or fears. It wouldn't have been fair. He just couldn't understand.

I had friends and family who were there to support me; they would listen and try to relate. But they couldn't. Part of the problem was that I struggled to put into words what I was really going through. At best, only a fraction of what was really going on inside of me ever came out in words. With only a partial story, they could do nothing but listen patiently, smile, and try to give advice and hope.

I truly could find no comfort, no one who really understood. I felt so alone.

As I lay on Jim's table, I told him this.

"It's like I am all alone in the middle of a barren wasteland. The wind is blowing and there's a sandstorm all around me. There is no one I can turn to. I can't see anyone and there isn't anyone who can see me. It's like there is only me and God."

Jim smiled and said, "Welcome to the real world."

The Real World

What is the real world anyway?

Aren't our families and home lives real? Aren't our jobs and responsibilities real? Friends, colleagues, and society—aren't they all real?

It isn't these actual people and things whose reality we have to question. It is our relationships with them that we have to look at.

When we are young, we look outside of ourselves to find security. We feel safe when we have a warm house, food on the table, and parents who care for us. These things define our world. They help us make decisions. Their existence makes the world make sense.

As we grow, we start to look a little wider for these things. We look to our extended family. We look to teachers, friends, colleagues, and ministers for advice and support. We look to belief systems to help make sense of the world. We look to larger institutions for our safety and security.

We believe in the institution of marriage—that this is something that we can count on for years of love and security. We believe that a good work ethic will always get us through the hard times.

We feel safe because the police force is there to control crime and the military will protect us from terrorism. There is the medical system whose doctors will fix us if we get sick and there is the church whose clergy will be there for our souls if we stray too far from the path.

We can often live a long time having full faith that we can depend on these things to help us out no matter what happens. We can depend on them for our safety, our happiness, and our peace of mind.

But what about the child whose parents are killed in a car crash? Or the woman whose husband leaves her for a younger woman after twenty-five years of marriage? Or the neighbourhood terrorized by crime lords? What about the people who died in the attack on the Twin Towers? Or the man who loses his job after thirty years when the plant shuts down? Or the person diagnosed with an "incurable" disease and sent home to die?

What about them?

What happened to their security and piece of mind?

The problem is that all of these things are just transitory. They all come and go throughout our lives. They are forever changing.

No matter how close we are to our loved ones, there will be times in our lives when they are with us and times when they are not. Parents die, children move out, people move away. Things change. People change. All of our relationships are temporary.

It is the same with our health. There will be times when it is good and times when it isn't. You could be healthy as a horse one day and sick in bed with the flu the next. You could have an accident and end up in the hospital with your whole life on hold. Or you could have a terminal illness and then, one day, the body starts to heal and you end up home and healthy for Christmas. You just never know.

When things like our health, our families, and our jobs are part of our security blanket, we are bound to have struggles in life, because by their nature, they aren't always going to be there. We are setting ourselves up for a fall.

We need to be able to feel secure. How can we do it if we can't count on the people and things around us?

EMBRACING AN UNPREDICTABLE WORLD

My suspicion is that the universe is not only queerer than we suppose, but queerer than we can suppose.
J. B. S. Haldane, Possible Worlds, 1927

In order to deal with this, we work hard at figuring out how the world works so that we can master it. Things may come and go, but maybe we can make sure that they come and go as *we* please.

We can do complicated calculations to figure out the movements of the planets and put people on the moon. We can construct great bridges using brilliant physics and engineering. We can sew people's legs back on and put dying people on life support.

Things like these give us a strange feeling of power and control over our universe. But is it real? Can we really predict the big things that go on around us? Do we actually have any control? Do we really have any idea what is going to happen tomorrow?

The truth is that we don't. We can guess. We can make predictions. In all likelihood, tomorrow will probably look a lot like today. But we really don't know. We tend not to like this reality. We want to know that if we do "A," then "B" will happen. We want a few rules to hedge our bets for the future.

This lack of comfort in an unpredictable future is something to be dealt with. This is where trust comes in. This is where you must ask yourself if you believe that this world is a friendly or an unfriendly place. Do you have faith in something bigger than you?

Can we handle not being able to control our world? Can we give up control and just trust that our inner guidance will lead us safely through?

GIVING UP CONTROL

Control is a double-sided issue when it comes to health because on the one hand, you have to take control of your life in order to get better and on the other hand, you have to let go of all control in everything else.

Many people with cancer feel like their life is out of their control. They feel like victims having been dealt a difficult blow. Their pecking order is all screwed up, so everyone around them is making all of their decisions for them. So, the first thing they need to do is take back that control. They need to get "Self" higher on their pecking order. They need to trust their inner feelings and wisdom that guide them on their path. They need to get their lives going in the direction of their dreams and hopes.

Then they have to give up all of that control by putting God on top of their pecking order. This loss of control feels different because at least it is a divine part of them that is in control, instead of the people around them. But as much as they are technically out of control, it isn't scary. They don't feel like a victim. They feel more like a player in a game waiting to see what is coming around the corner. There is more excitement and less hand-wringing.

CONTROL AND PSALM 23

Giving up this control can be a challenge. But does this sense of control actually make us feel happy? Does it really make us feel secure? I wonder about that.

One winter day, I was driving to work. I lived out in the country and the roads were really icy and snow-covered. At one point, I was heading down a steep hill and I lost control of my car. I tried to correct and counter-steer but I was on a sheet of ice. There was nothing I could do.

I realized that I might die. But I also realized that I had no control over that, and then the strangest thing happened. Time seemed to slow down. I felt no fear. I was completely peaceful. I wasn't even afraid of dying.

I put one hand on the steering wheel and one hand on my stomach (I was six months pregnant at the time), and I closed my eyes. The car careened off the road, over an eight-foot drop, hit a fencepost in midair, and landed in a farmer's field. Once the car stopped moving, I opened my eyes. The windshield was completely smashed. The crumple zone at the front of the car was completely crumpled. And the car was actually still running. I sat there for a moment amazed that I was still alive and extremely grateful. Then I turned the car off, got into a passing truck, which took me home, jumped into my in-laws' K-car, and headed off to work again.

The experience didn't even shake me. I had no fear attached to it at all. It amazed me how calm and serene the whole experience had been.

Then, a few days later, I heard someone on the radio talking about Psalm 23. He said it was all about letting go of control in your life and feeling the overwhelming peace that brings.

> The Lord is my shepherd; I shall not want
> He maketh me to lie down in green pastures: he leadeth me beside the still waters.
> He restoreth my soul: he leadeth me in the paths of righteousness for his name's sake.
> Yea, though I walk through the valley of the shadow of death, I will fear no evil: for thou art with me; thy rod and thy staff they comfort me.
> Thou preparest a table before me in the presence of mine enemies: thou anointest my head with oil; my cup runneth over.
> Surely goodness and mercy shall follow me all the days of my life; and I will dwell in the house of the Lord forever.

In the car that day, there was a point where I realized that I had no control over the situation. At that point, I left my fate to God. God became my shepherd. My experience became the peace that one feels when lying down in green pastures beside still waters. Yea, though I was flying through the air into a fence post, I feared no evil. I was comforted. And although death was a possibility, I was blissfully happy.

And what about the goodness and mercy that will follow me for the rest of my life? Well, the greatest thing I gained was the experience, knowing that that kind of peace is possible even in dire straits. That is a phenomenal peace to carry with you.

As it turns out, my experience was not unique. Six months later, my father-in-law was driving a tractor hauling a wagon of beans to the local mill. As he headed down a steep hill, part of the steering mechanism of the tractor seized and he had no control of the tractor. The tractor went flying down the hill, off the road, and into the swamp, with the ten-ton load of soybeans pressing the tractor and my father-in-law down into the muck.

Miraculously, the back window of the tractor opened. It had been jammed shut for years. He slipped out of the tractor and started walking home.

Well, my mother-in-law was out of her mind. She was horrified at what could've happened. Most of the neighbourhood turned out at my in-laws' place to drink coffee, hear the story, and congratulate my father-in-law on still being there to talk about it. Every relative, neighbour, and friend was there talking, telling stories of other close calls, fretting, or comforting my mother-in-law.

As I watched the crazy scene, I noticed my father-in-law over in a corner of the room just sitting pretty quietly. Most assumed that he was just shaken from the accident and being quiet. I had other suspicions.

So I went over to sit beside him and asked him, "So, how did you feel when you realized that you had no control over the tractor?"

He looked at me for a moment and then said, "You know, it's the strangest thing. Once I realized that I couldn't do anything, I was completely calm. I wasn't afraid at all."

I said, "I know exactly what you mean."

Looking Inside for Reality

We don't really want the control. We think we do, but it is only our brains. All we really want to know is that we'll be okay.

In those moments when I was in the car and I knew that I was not in control, I was truly happy—happier than I had ever been. I had no stresses. I had no worries. Even though my life was in danger, I was completely at peace.

Imagine living like that every day. Imagine being so sure that everything was fine, that you never had to worry or stress about anything. I think that this is the true leap of faith. I think that we can truly live like that. I think that that is the point of Psalm 23. We just have to be willing to try it.

It is a lot like riding a roller coaster. No matter how crazy the ride is, if we trust that the safety harnesses will keep us safely in the seat then we can relax and enjoy the ride.

But if we aren't sure if the ride is safe and we don't think that the harnesses will hold us in, then how can we possibly enjoy the ride? How can we be anything but terrified the whole time?

The only security that we truly have is inside of us. It is the knowledge that we are connected to something greater. It is knowing that there is always guidance waiting for us if we want it. It is knowing that, one way or another, everything will be okay.

In the end, the only constant, dependable realities are ourselves and God. Everyone and everything else will come and go. We will have relationships, jobs, and different circumstances. But the common thread will always be us and our inner voice.

That connection is our only real security blanket. It is the only thing that we can always depend on to help make our decisions. It is the only thing that will always be there. It is the only thing that can ever give us true peace of mind.

Chapter Seventeen
The Day Before the Lump Left

The decision you make may not be right for another person on this planet. But it will be right for you.

Jim

I woke up the next morning in terrible pain.

By this time, the lump was pushing about half an inch out of the side of my breast and was really painful. It hurt to walk. It hurt to move. I didn't know what to do. I couldn't really take care of the kids. I couldn't really take care of me. I was getting really tired. Deep down, I knew I was on the right path, but in moments like this I was definitely losing some faith in the process.

My dad offered to take care of the kids for a while, until I was feeling better. I hoped maybe a week would do it. But I really didn't know. I was really thankful because I found it doubly hard to sort out everything Jim was telling me with the kids around.

I would be deep in thought about something that he had said and inevitably one of the kids would need me. They were two and four years old. I could expect nothing less. But it was really hard on the healing process.

Soon after the kids had gone with their grandparents, I went for an appointment with Jim. As I lay on his table, all of my defences came down. I started crying. I suddenly realized just how tired I was. I realized how much I didn't want to be in pain anymore. I was struggling to know if I was doing the right thing. The fatigue was really wearing down my resolve.

I looked at Jim and said, "Jim, what would you do if you were me?"

"If I were you, I'd go and get that thing cut out of there. I wouldn't walk around in as much pain as you are in!"

And I cried, "But I don't want to get it cut out. That's not what I'm supposed to do. That's not the way!"

"Then that's all you need to know. The decision you make may not be right for another person on this planet. But it will be right for you."

Those words would ring in my ears many, many times. It became an absolute truth for me—that any decision only has to be right for me, not anyone else on the planet. It freed me forever of worrying about what anyone else thought of anything I did, dreamt, or hoped for.

NO SIMPLE EQUATION FOR HEALING

The cure for cancer is different for every person.

We like simple answers. We like formulas. We like A + B = C. Simple makes us feel safer. But the cure for cancer is not a simple linear equation. There is no equation that says, "No Sweets + More Broccoli + Breastfeed Babies + Chemotherapy = Cure for Cancer." There just isn't any such equation.

We are not simple machines that require simple solutions. We are infinitely complex living beings that require dynamic and unique solutions.

People would ask me what I did to get better. They hoped that maybe if they did what I did, then they could get well too. The problem is that I can't tell anyone what they need to do to stay healthy or to cure themselves of whatever is ailing them.

The reality is that we were all created differently. We are individuals. We are each here to experience this world through our own specific and unique perspectives.

None of us is in the same situation. No one else has our genetics, upbringing, stresses, intelligence, emotions, diet, optimism, depression, relationships, and current situation. Every aspect of who we are is unique. And the combination of all of these things truly creates a unique situation.

Each of us has our own path to take. And therefore, we each are given specific guidance that is just for us. So, even though there might be aspects of our lives that seem similar—family histories, strange lumps, and similar diagnoses—we still have to honour the path that brought us to this point. And for each of us it was different.

We must find our own unique healthy life equation. It might be taking up yoga or becoming a vegetarian or getting Reiki treatments. It might be surgery, radiation, and chemotherapy. Or it might be drinking beer and watching bad B-movies every Saturday night with our friends. Whatever it is, it is the process of finding it and living it that will make us healthy and happy.

In the process of finding this equation, we will find out what makes us tick. We will take control of our lives, honour our body's wisdom, listen to our intuition, and have faith in the process. Our resulting journeys might all look different. But the process is the same for everyone.

ONLY ONE STEP AT A TIME

Trusting your inner self to map out your road to wellness can be a little daunting. It can feel like a monumental and nearly impossible task to take on. But all we need is "just enough light for the step we're on."

We can only figure out our personal equation one step at a time. This is because every time we make a decision, everything changes. Every choice causes a ripple effect throughout our lives and those of others. If we make a different choice, then a different ripple is caused.

Let's say that you feel called to take a yoga class once a week. Imagine that you end up friends with the woman who stretches beside you each week, and she goes to this great chiropractor who also does acupuncture. You then choose to go and check this guy out. Between the treatments and a new tea you are drinking, your longstanding lower-back pain is finally gone. Because of this, you decide that you want to start bicycling regularly because you love biking but haven't been able to do so because of your bad back. And so on.

This is why we can't always know what the second step is until we have taken the first step. After the first step, things are different. We have to see how things shake out after the first decision. Then we can assess our new situation and contemplate the next step.

Although we are trained that we have to figure out the whole situation right now, that just isn't how life actually works. Our lives are constantly changing. Things are in constant flux.

This is where being able to listen for the guidance all of the time is so valuable—where you truly live in the moment because you know that your circumstances are always changing. This is what it is to truly live on the edge, where life gets really interesting, where you get to live completely in the present.

This is where you feel vital and alive!

Chapter Eighteen
Miracles

Miracles are not contrary to nature, but only contrary to what we know about nature.

St. Augustine

This particular morning wasn't really any more interesting than any other.

Physically, I felt the same as I had felt most days. The lump had moved quite a bit now and was jutting out about an inch from the edge of my breast. There were shock waves running through my body most of the time, which was very strange but not scary. I was tired but fine.

After having breakfast, I decided to have a bath.

This was no small decision, because getting in and out of the bathtub was an ordeal in itself. Since my breast hurt no matter which way I moved, it required ridiculous contortions to simply get in and out of the bathtub.

Once settled in the bath, I relaxed. There was no pain—just heat, steam, and relaxation. It was truly wonderful.

I'd like to say that I had a great revelation at that moment that made the next few minutes make sense. But I didn't. It was a pretty typical bath. Afterward I worked myself to a standing position in order to shower off.

I was about to turn on the shower when I had the strangest feeling in my breast. As I looked down, a small hole had appeared in the edge of the lump and stuff was coming out of it. What was coming out was a combination of pus, blood, clear fluids, and solids. It just pulsed out of me at a very steady rate. The pain was gone. The body shocks were gone.

As the fluids continued to pulse out of my breast, my mind was in a completely different place. Some would call it nirvana. Some might call it a delta brain state. Some would call it heaven. I don't know what it was. But I do know that it was wonderful. It was a feeling of complete bliss.

It felt like I wasn't even part of this world. If someone had walked into the bathroom, I'm not sure that I could even have spoken to them. I simply wasn't there. I just stood there and floated on a cloud while the fluid and material flowed out of me.

I stood there for three hours. That seems like a ludicrous amount of time now. But in those moments, time truly stood still. I just stood there until the pulsing stopped and nothing more came out.

When I stepped out of the bathtub, I was completely free of pain! There was a gaping hole in my breast where the lump had been. But I was beyond joyous. I was ecstatic. I yelled out the window to my husband, "The lump is gone! The lump is gone!"

The elation I felt was unbelievable. I was so glad it was over. I was so glad to be free of pain. I was utterly amazed at what had happened. It was one of those indescribable moments that words just don't do justice.

It was especially wonderful after months of trying to hear and follow my inner voice. Most of the time, I felt that I was doing the right thing at each step. But there was always some doubt about whether I was making the right decisions. Sometimes the doubt came from other people. But most of the time it came from me, especially when I was unclear as to what I needed to do next.

The lump leaving like this was like a warm hug after running a marathon, and it gave me a huge sense of satisfaction. I had followed my heart and it had turned out really well. This was absolutely the greatest thing that I took away from this experience. I had followed my heart. There was no one to look to for help in my decisions. It had just been between me and God. And now the lump was gone. It was a great end to a challenging time.

One curious thing about the time that I stood in the shower was the thoughts that kept running through my mind. For the entire three hours, the phrase "By the grace of God" repeated over and over. I wasn't consciously thinking it. That phrase was just running itself over and over again. Truthfully, I didn't know what to think of it. Mostly I was just extremely thankful.

The only meaning that I could guess at was that I was not to own this victory. I was not to go shouting from the rooftops, "I cured myself of cancer!" This was very clear to me. In fact, when people would ask me how I did it, I could honestly tell them that I didn't really know. I knew that I had played a part. But I wasn't alone in it. I couldn't own it all.

Later, I called Jim to tell him what had happened. He was thrilled. I thanked him endlessly for all of his help, and I told him that I absolutely couldn't have done it without him.

Jim got quiet and then he said, "I have to tell you something."

"Okay."

"I didn't do anything. You did it all."

"What do you mean? There were all of those appointments and treatments. You were doing stuff. I saw you."

"Oh, I did some massage work and we talked a lot. But I was never allowed to heal you. You see, when I work with someone, I do it through prayer. I ask what they need and I am told what to do. Sometimes, I am told to put my hands here and there, and the lumps in the body completely disappear. But with you, every time I asked, I got a very strong 'No—don't touch her.' It was very strange. That's why we spent most of the time talking. You were meant to do this on your own. I don't know why."

I didn't know what to say to that. So, we just chatted about how I felt when the lump was leaving and he advised me to just keep some gauze over the hole until it was healed.

The hole seeped for about three weeks. It seemed to heal from the inside out. Today, there is no scar—no sign of the previous battle. If you dig down into the breast tissue, you can tell that there is a bit of a hole where something once took up space, but it is nothing noticeable.

The other interesting outcome is that there was no matting in my breasts anymore. The matting that was endemic in my family was all gone. And I have never had any more since.

WHAT IS A MIRACLE?

What happened to me felt like a miracle. It was beyond my understanding. It went beyond logic and reason. It just felt miraculous.

When we are diagnosed with a serious illness, we seldom consider the occurrence of a miracle as one of the possible outcomes. The chances are so slim, why would we get our hopes up?

But what is a miracle, anyway? The Collins Dictionary tells us that the word itself comes from the Latin word *miraculum*, which is from the root word *mirari*, "to wonder at." Essentially, that is the definition of a miracle—anything that we wonder at. A closer look at the dictionary reveals another definition—"an event contrary to the laws of nature and attributed to a supernatural cause."

Miracles are simply happenings that don't follow our observed and defined laws of nature. They aren't strange or odd or unlikely. They are just outside our current understanding—outside our current theory of what is possible.

We create scientific theories to help us define what we observe all around us. We have sciences to describe what we see happening inside our bodies. We have sciences that describe the weather, animals, plants, rocks, and the oceans. We have sciences that describe how different forces affect each other and how different chemicals interact.

But all scientific theories are simply our best guesses based on what we have observed up until this point. As soon as something happens that doesn't fit with the theory, then the theory must be looked at and revised, or scrapped altogether.

It's like the theory that the Earth was flat or that it was the centre of the universe. These theories were taken as absolute scientific fact for centuries until a number of scientists produced evidence that they were in fact incorrect.

Miracles are the kinds of things that don't fit into current theories. They simply don't follow the laws that we have laid out thus far. They are the people who survive after being given only six weeks to live. They are the people who walk away from total car wrecks with only a couple of scratches. They are the people who survived their troubled youth, against all odds.

Sceptics call them flukes. Believers call them acts of God. But regardless of what you call them, the reality is that they happen. And they happen all of the time. The problem is that when we call them flukes or acts of God, we create the idea that they aren't normal—that they aren't a common part of everyday life.

If they were flukes, then there was just a blip in the system. It isn't really possible. It was an error in the process. If they are considered an act of God, then this also is outside of our normal possibilities because we had to be in God's good graces in order to have this gift bestowed upon us. It was just divine intervention, or in other words, an other-worldly experience.

The problem is that both of these situations put the idea of healing spontaneously outside of our control and outside of our normal set of possibilities.

But what if living with miracles is actually supposed to be normal?

Is it so impossible to imagine that we could live in a world we could wonder at? Could we not have a balance between understanding certain things and allowing other things to be beyond our comprehension?

Einstein once said that "there are only two ways to live your life. One is as though nothing is a miracle. The other is as though everything is a miracle." He was clear that there were certain aspects of our world that were comprehensible and others that were simply miraculous. And he was one of the greatest scientific minds of our lifetime!

Miracles and Our Health

Believing in miracles is simply the openness to allow something to happen that we might not understand. Being open to this is huge in the land of being healthy and recovering from illness.

When we honour our pecking order and listen to that little voice inside, we don't necessarily know what will happen next. We haven't calculated it and done the proper research. We are just trusting that divine part of us and going forward.

When we do this, we are opening ourselves up for a miracle. We are opening ourselves up for something new, something that we couldn't have come up with on our own, something beyond our current understanding.

This applies whether it is the common cold that we want to get rid of, whether we are trying to get pregnant, whether we are hospitalized with a serious illness, or we just don't want to get cancer. At any point, listening to that wisdom within always opens that door to the miraculous—to an alternate path to the known.

Believing in miracles means not having to overthink. It means being able to see the world through the eyes of a child. It means taking things as they come without analysis and expectation.

It means that regardless of all the studies, your family history, and everything that you've ever heard, anything is still possible. Statistics are just a numbers game. They are not real life. What happens next in your life depends on your choices right now. And regardless of how smart we think we are, we have no idea what that future will be.

It could be something expected. Or it could be a miracle.

Chapter Nineteen
The Birth of This Book

A few years after the lump had disappeared, I found myself in the bank talking to a woman about getting a loan. Somehow, we got to talking about the fact that she had had breast cancer a few years before. She had gone through chemotherapy, radiation, and the whole bit. As she shared with me how it had changed her life, I was shocked to realize how similar the changes in our lives were.

She told me how she now was a lot more careful about what she agreed to do for people. She now had a voice that she previously didn't. She spent more time doing things that she enjoyed. She cared a lot less about what other people thought and listened a lot more to her own inner promptings.

She could have been reading out of my diary. I had made all of the changes in my life that she had. I shared her "aha" moments.

Here we were, two women with family histories of breast cancer having gone entirely different routes. Hers was medical and mine was alternative. And yet, we came up with the same results.

Was this just a coincidence? Was it just a fluke that we could start in similar places and then end up in the same place, despite the fact that what happened in between was so radically different?

I wondered if other people who had healed from cancer had also made similar changes. So, I started researching other healings, spontaneous remissions, healings against the odds, etc.

What I found was that the stories were very similar—people having "aha" moments, people starting to live their own lives, people no longer caring about what other people think of them, people finding God, people finding and enjoying their gifts. But mostly, people finding a real reason to live and enjoy life.

That was the birth of this book.

I thought, "What if you could skip the cancer?" What if you didn't have to go through the crisis of cancer and just skip to the end lesson? What if you could learn from all of these people's experiences? What if there were changes that you could make in your life today that mirror the changes required for a miraculous healing?

Could you learn the lessons first and skip the cancer?

I believe that the answer is a resounding *yes!*

WHERE DO WE GO FROM HERE?

Cancer is not easy. Even after everything that I have been through, the idea that I might have breast cancer still brings fear to my heart. But it isn't the fear of the disease, and it isn't the fear of dying.

It is the fear of the changes that might be needed in my life to get through it. It is the idea that maybe I am still lying to myself about how happy I really am. Am I still saying yes to people when my heart is saying no? Am I walking my talk and truly living from an intuitive place? Do I have a truly healthy relationship with my husband and kids? Or am I still fooling myself?

These are not easy questions. And because they are basically the stuff of my everyday life, the idea of changing them still strikes a chord of fear within me.

But it isn't the cancer I fear anymore. Cancer is just the knock on the door that says, "It's time to wake up! It's time to live your *real* life! Change is a-coming!"

And so, if the idea of making these changes makes you afraid, please know that it did for me too—and it still does! I don't want to pretend that it is easy to change how you see yourself and how you interact with your loved ones. It's not.

But, as difficult as it is, things truly are better, happier, and more fulfilling in the end.

And so I ask you to have hope and courage. Change is the hardest thing. It is much harder than cancer. But it is worth it.

Your fear of cancer is your opportunity to make changes. This is your chance. It is often only through necessity that we make real changes. And you can start right now.

It doesn't matter what your past has been. Each day is a new day.

It doesn't matter what choices you've made in the past. You can make new ones today.

Feel free to re-create your life. Feel free to start clean now.
Be honest. Walk in truth. Be healthy.
See what happens.

We are reading the first verse of the first chapter of a book
whose pages are infinite.
Author unknown

REFERENCE LIST

Below is a partial list of books that inspired me while I was researching this book. A full bibliography of books, journal articles, magazines and case studies would take over ten pages to print, and it wouldn't really be that interesting. My original manuscript was filled with facts and figures having to do with the healing process, but in the revision process, we found that they didn't fit anywhere. Perhaps they are not what helps us make the big changes in our lives—perhaps it is the stories themselves that really make the difference.

You might ask why are there so many books on chaos theory and quantum physics in this list. As I began researching people who had healed, I wanted to have some understanding about *how* these things happened. I found that these sciences hold the framework that we need to understand our phenomenally complex minds, bodies, and spirits.

Chopra, Deepak. *Quantum Healing: Exploring the Frontiers of Mind/ Body Medicine*. Bantam Books. New York. 1989

Cousins, Norman. *Anatomy of an Illness*. Bantam Books. New York. 1979.

Covey, Stephen. *The 7 Habits of Highly Effective People*. Free Press. New York. 2003.

Ferguson, Marilyn. *Aquarius Now*. Weiser Books. Boston. 2005.

Frankl, Viktor E. *Man's Search for Meaning*. Simon & Schuster. New York. 1984.

Gleick, James. *Chaos: Making a New Science*. Penguin Books. New York. 1987.

Goldstien, Jan. *Life Can Be This Good: Awakening to the Miracles All Around Us*. Conari Press. Berkeley, California. 2002.

Hawkins, David. *Power vs. Force.* Hay House. Carlsbad, California. 1995.

Jung, C.G. *Modern Man in Search of a Soul.* Routledge and Kegan Paul, Ltd. London. 1933.

LeShan, Lawrence. *Cancer as a Turning Point: A Handbook for People With Cancer, Their Families, and Health Professionals.* Fitzhenry & Whiteside. Toronto. 1989.

Lewis, C. S. *The Horse and His Boy.* Scholastic, Inc. New York. 1954.

Lorenz, Edward N. *The Essence of Chaos.* University of Washington Press. Seattle. 1993.

May, Rollo. *The Discovery of Being: Writings in Existential Psychology.* W.W. Norton & Company. New York. 1983

Myss, Caroline. *Anatomy of the Spirit.* Crown Publishers. New York. 1996.

Ouspensky, P. D. *In Search of the Miraculous.* Harcourt, Inc. Orlando, Florida. 1949.

Pagels, Heinz R. *The Cosmic Code: Quantum Physics as the Language of Nature.* Michael Joseph. London. 1983.

Pert, Candace B. *Molecules of Emotion.* Scribner. New York. 1997.

Prigonine, Ilya, and Isabelle Stengers. *Order Out of Chaos: Man's New Dialogue With Nature.* Bantam Books. New York. 1984.

Schachter-Shalomi, Zalman. *From Age-ing to Sage-ing.* Warner Books. New York. 1995.

Siegel, Bernie. *Peace, Love & Healing.* Harper & Row Publishers. New York. 1989.

Simonton, O. Carl. and Reid Henson with Brenda Hampton. *The Healing Journey.* Authors Choice Press. Lincoln, Nebraska. 1992.

Simonton, O. Carl, Stephanie Matthews-Simonton, and James L. Creighton. *Getting Well Again.* Bantam Books. Toronto. 1978.

Waldrop, M. Mitchell. *Complexity: The Emerging Science at the Edge of Order and Chaos.* Simon & Schuster. New York. 1992.

ACKNOWLEDGMENTS

I now join the long list of authors who just cannot thank their editor enough. Without Ryan Schrauben, this book would not be what it is. After all of the edits, deletions, and rewrites, there were many times that I wondered if there would be anything left. Were we editing the soul out of it? Would it even sound like me in the end? But the book turned out just how I wanted—honest, helpful, and to the point (which is nothing short of a miracle some days when you're as long-winded as I am). So, thank you Ryan, for your kindness, your patience, and your wonderful, good advice.

I want to thank Marian Nelson of Nelson Publishing & Marketing for believing that this book was worth publishing. You provide a unique and wonderful opportunity for authors—access to a professional team who create great books, and the ability to be a part of every step in the process. Thank you for valuing that the author's voice must always come through. But most of all, thank you Marian for your kindness and your unending support.

I would like to thank Jim. I know you won't like this, but I truly consider you my first guru—someone I could really trust who taught me the wisdom that I needed. Thank you for raising the bar in every aspect of my life. Thank you Jim, for your friendship. Thanks for everything.

And finally, I would like to thank my beautiful family and wonderful friends. Thank you for always encouraging me to tell my story and to get this book published. But most of all, thank you for showing me that unconditional love is real and possible. Thank you for loving me even when I am my true, quirky self (and for loving me all those years when I wasn't). To my family and friends, thank you, thank you, thank you.

ABOUT THE AUTHOR

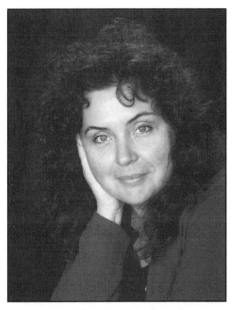

Katrina Bos was born in Toronto, Ontario, and originally studied mathematics at the University of Waterloo. As the eldest child of two teachers, and with a natural inclination toward academia, it was easy for Katrina to become a bit of an intellectual and an idealist. Five years of studying university mathematics further ingrained in her the ability to "live in one's head" and the notion that anything could be sorted out on paper.

Soon after graduation, she married a farmer and moved to rural Ontario. Getting married, moving to the country, and having children turned out to be just the grounding experience that this intellectual and idealist needed. Milking cows, the struggles of isolation, and the natural challenges of marriage and raising children soon threw all of her ideals and well-laid plans out the window.

For Katrina, a more intuitive, heartfelt approach seemed to be the only way through. She returned to university to study psychology, family, and religious studies. She began doing counselling work and writing uplifting columns for several local newspapers. She opened a dance studio and studied Kundalini yoga.

Today, she teaches classes in yoga, meditation, and dance. A fun and engaging public speaker, she gives talks on topics that uplift the human spirit and lead to a greater understanding of what life is all about. She currently lives near Goderich, Ontario, with her husband, two children, two dogs, two horses, assorted cats, and a few hundred cows.

For additional information, please visit www.katrinabos.ca.